Hidden Data:

The Blind Eye of Science

Helene Z. Hill

West Orange, NJ

To Dr. Gordon Sato
One of the few people I know for whom
integrity is a middle name.
  Lanie Hill

Cover photo: collection of Helene Z. Hill. This photograph was taken on March 29, 2001. See Chapter 12, page 69. 100 mm tissue culture dishes numbers 1 and 7 were inoculated each with a tiny sample taken from experimental Helena tubes numbers 1 and 7 and incubated overnight at 37 degrees centigrade. The observed cloudiness that developed was due to the presence of rod shaped bacteria observed microscopically. The control dish (K) contained uninoculated medium alone. No bacteria were observed.

Figure 1 © Genetics Society of America
Figures 10 and 12 © American Association for Cancer Research
Figure 11 © Springer
Figure 13 Left © Oxford University Press
Figures 13 Right and 15 © Elsevier
Figure 14 © John Wiley and Sons
Figure 16 2 upper gels © Springer
Figure 16 Lower gel © John Wiley and Sons

HillTree Farm Press
Printed by CreateSpace, North Charleston, South Carolina

Praise for Hidden Data

The current system of science misconduct adjudication in the United States, often indifferent to scientific evidence, is broken. Competing interests abound at universities and honest reporting is a casualty. The painstakingly detailed presentation of statistical evidence of data manipulation by Dr. Hill is an example of the Herculean efforts that some scientists are forced to undertake, in opposition to institutions, in order to tell the truth. That an honest investigator should feel compelled to labor in this way is a tragedy. You can read it here.

Bart Kahr, Ph.D.
Professor of Chemistry
New York University

Hill presents convincing evidence for scientific misconduct by a former colleague and chronicles her long struggle to bring this evidence to light. She also succeeds in reviewing the problem of fraud in science and the importance of statistical analysis in the detection of fraud.

Brian Palestis, Ph.D.
Professor and Chair, Biological Sciences
Wagner College

Whistle-blowers want science fraud to be punished. The bioscience establishment wishes fraud would disappear. Helene Hill's research was damaged by a fraud, and for more than 15 years the establishment's fraud police have fought to keep the fraud hidden.

Charles W. McCutchen, Ph.D.
Physicist, Inventor

Helene was there before there was a there

Clare Francis
Whistle blower

Hidden Data is a courageous look at how the enterprise of science is corrupted by a lack of integrity. We all suffer when individual and institutional status takes precedence over truth. Dr. Hill's story chronicles a journey too few scientists are willing to take. Hidden Data is a wake-up call to all of us. Something needs to be done. Hidden Data should be mandatory reading for every budding scientist.

Sigrid Fry-Revere, J.D., Ph.D.
President, Center for Ethical Solutions

Dr. Hill presents a compelling argument to demonstrate that Courts faced with claims of fraud in scientific research and the grant writing process should not be allowed to view them as an exception to, rather than directly actionable under the Federal False Claims Act and other State Whistleblower Laws. Conflicting data that is the result of fabrication may well rise to the level of research misconduct that mandates a Court take seriously the implications for public health.

Sheldon H. Pincus, Esq
Bucceri and Pincus, Esqs

In religion one can often be forgiven for one's sins, but no one should be forgiven for sins against science.

Kendric C. Smith, Ph.D.
Professor Emeritus, Radiation Biology
Stanford University School of Medicine

This is a harrowing story that spanned many years. It is about human, institutional and societal failure in the scientific world. Data was falsified; institutional cover up took place and the judicial system could not unravel the truth. How could this fate possibly befall the highly recognized and respected professor who taught me the baby steps of the scientific method? The truth is that corrupting forces pervade and it is when falsehood runs up against the strength of someone like Dr. Hill that good prevails.

The damaging effect of scientific fraud and intellectual dishonesty is for all to see: Vioxx deaths, measles resurgence and false stem cell hopes. Dr. Hill meticulously described her courageous and relentless battle against massive negative forces. Ironically she also skillfully used the scientific method to bring out the truth. It is a reminder that honor and scientific honesty is priceless. This book should interest all those seeking the truth. This is especially true for those involved in public and academic policies. Hopefully history will not be allowed to repeat itself and that in the end, public interest will be well served. I personally am most fortunate and thankful to have been in the tutelage of Dr. Hill.

Frank K. Kwong M.D.
Former Allergy Consultant, The White House
Allergy & Immunology Consultant, Cedars Sinai Medical Center, UCLA
Allergy & Immunology Consultant, Greater Los Angeles VA Medical System, UCLA

This is the remarkable story of a brave scientist, the price she paid for her bravery, and the reaction of the academic establishment to her allegations of research misconduct. Today scientists in training, if funded by the NIH or the NSF, are required under federal law to receive formal instruction in the responsible conduct of research (RCR). Helene Hill's book, and the lessons it teaches, should be part of their training.

Danielle Brian, Executive Director
Ned Feder, M.D, Staff Scientist
Project On Government Oversight

Dr. Helene Hill's courageous book illustrates the ethical dilemma that all whistleblowers face: Seeking the truth is dangerous! I know first-hand because I too am a whistleblower. Dr. Hill's book is an insightful guide to doing what's right even under the most damaging and frightful actions of others. Thank you Dr. Hill for your remarkable book and for exposing the misconduct. Your integrity and pursuit of the truth is inspiring.

Amy Block Joy, Ph.D. Emeritus, University of California and author of **Whistleblower** and **Retaliation**

There are a surprising and troubling number of U.S. researchers who have had experiences similar to Professor Hill's. She and I often remark to each other on the similarities of our whistle-blower experiences: the widespread turning a blind eye to misconduct and the willful failures by responsible institutions and federal agencies to adequately investigate, if there is any investigation at all. We share the further experience of having taken our claims to court, which all too often, at best, allows the recovery of additional evidence of misconduct. There are whistle-blowers with whom I have dealt who have had the discovery phase of their legal action completely blocked, in what seems to have been the opposite of a pursuit of justice in our courts.

Most whistle-blowers I know are very determined people and are often relentless in hunting down evidence relevant to their cases. This certainly includes Professor Hill. However, even when presented with "smoking gun" quality information indicating that investigation is warranted, academic institutions, scientific journals, and other responsible parties remain remarkably resistant to act appropriately, despite proclaiming publicly that they adhere to various ethical standards. Indeed, in my experience, successful whistle-blowers are less defined by the quality of the evidence they obtain in support of allegations than by the publicity they, or journalists who happen to take an interest in their cases, generate. Dr. Hill is among the most publicly driven of all the whistleblowers that I have worked with in recent years. This book, which I had the pleasure of reading and commenting on in earlier versions, is more evidence of Dr. Hill's relentless push to get information out about her experience with serious flaws in the handling of allegations of research misconduct in the U.S. I hope that this work helps produce a step forward in improving that process.

Robert Bauchwitz M.D., Ph.D.

The subtlety of scientific misrepresentation is carefully documented in this book. The statistical analysis backs up simple observation of how sloppy science is conducted. The problem outlined here is so pervasive that some readers may hardly see anything surprising or disturbing. However, hidden data should surprise and disturb anyone who cares about science.

Stefan Franzen, Ph.D.
Professor
Biophysical and Biological Chemistry
North Carolina State University

Helene Hill depicts the characteristics of an absolutist who follows her conscience for the good of the citizens.

Don Ray Soeken, LCSW-C, Ph.D.
Author, Psychiatric Social Worker

Dr. Margot O'Toole speaks out

Helene Hill and I share two life-altering experiences - reporting clear evidence of scientific misconduct and discovering that the academic establishment does not care to deal with it. In my case, independent review by an expert panel of scientists set up by the Office of Research Integrity - which reviews cases involving government funded research - found in my favor. The expert panel overturned a cover up by a university internal review and, based on overwhelming scientific evidence, returned a finding of misconduct (https://ori.hhs.gov/images/ddblock/vol3_no1.pdf). However, the scientist who was found by the expert scientific panel to have committed misconduct, pushed on under a legal framework with appeal and obtained a reversal before the Appeals Board of the Department of Health and Human Services (https://ori.hhs.gov/images/ddblock/vol4_no4.pdf). Scientists and non-scientists who stand outside the circle of any particular case understandably assume that the final disposition of a case should be accepted as trustworthy. And what logical argument can those of us who are whistleblowers offer against this reasonable assumption, especially when we are dealing with science, an endeavor whose primary guiding principle is to explore and report accurately? After pondering this challenge for the last 30 years, I see extraordinarily strong similarities between the worldwide sexual abuse scandal in the Catholic Church (which is now universally acknowledged to have been a reality), and scientific misconduct in academia (in which issues raised by a few pesky whistleblowers are widely regarded as unimportant abnormalities). In both scientific and Catholic Church communities the fundamental mission represents two of the highest human aspirations – the church promoting selfless service to others and science pushing to advance knowledge for the benefit of all mankind. In both communities, insiders who receive and adjudicate allegations are themselves almost certainly passionately committed to the mission. Under these circumstances, reactions of covering up or circling the wagons might strike such insiders as justifiable in any individual case. For example, I was told that science is 99.99% pure, and insisting on correction of just one published article would only endanger funding and careers. In the case of the Catholic Church, protecting the larger mission of the church was the rationale for covering up for individual abusive priests. It is now well established that the Church's policy of covering up resulted in a worldwide epidemic of child abuse. In the scientific community, we are at the point where a very few among us, with Helene Hill front and center, have brought forward unwelcome evidence. The establishment responses are based on the premise that this great and important endeavor is fundamentally sound - and therefore the treatment of whistleblowers and the disposition of their cases should be of little or no concern. Failure to deal with misconduct leaves this noble human endeavor, in fact all endeavors, vulnerable to the spread of corruption. When review processes are ineffective, inaccurate or inappropriate they serve only as a license to the community at large to move along without further concern. In science the attitude should be, as it should have been in the Catholic Church, that we protect our mission against corruption because tolerated corruption becomes pervasive corruption. Helene Hill has my admiration for grasping the importance of this fundamental principle and taking such extraordinary measures to shine light on attitudes to corruption within the scientific community.

Margot O'Toole, Ph.D.

Dedication

To my husband, George, who has stood by me through thick and thin, to my family, who hold the future in their hands. May they always remember that the pathways of truth are the easiest to follow. And to the myriad honest scientists out there – may they be the ones to light the way.

I have a right to be blind sometimes

Vice Admiral Horatio Nelson

The lie was dead and damned, and truth stood up instead

Robert Browning

HIDDEN DATA

FOREWORD

If the history books *get it right*, Helene Z. Hill will be remembered as a scientist ahead of her time. Typically such accolades are afforded to Nobel Prize winners and others who make ground-breaking discoveries. In Dr. Hill's case, her efforts to shine light onto the dark underbelly of scientific misconduct began at a time when nobody else was even considering such things could happen.

Hill's story begins in the late 1990s when the number of publicly known misconduct cases in the academic sciences could be counted on the digits of one hand. It ends in 2011 and encompasses a decade during which the ground shifted beneath our feet, in terms of how science deals with misconduct. In the last five years, the pace has quickened further, and with the help of the Internet, there are fewer and fewer opportunities for less-than-honorable scientists to continue operating un-exposed.

I was honored to be asked to write this foreword, because although my experiences in this area have not been nearly as long-term or emotionally wrenching as Hill's, some key characteristics are similar. In 2012, I started a blog (www.science-fraud.org) aimed at highlighting irregularities in life science publications, mostly involving re-use of figures and data. Over the course of its brief existence, the blog reported on 275 papers, before a barrage of legal threats forced its closure in early 2013. Although my University faculty position was tenured, and I did not lose my job over the affair, the University refused legal support and I was forced to pay a local law firm several thousand dollars from my own pocket to defend against blusterous threats from disgruntled scientists whose work was reported on. Just like the tens of thousands of dollars Hill spent on her own failed legal case, that money is gone forever, with the only real winners being the lawyers who encourage litigation in such matters. It is somewhat telling that, of those who threatened to sue me, two have lost their jobs (one has filed suit against their employer for wrongful dismissal), one was exonerated by a highly suspicious (and possibly corrupt) local investigation panel, and all have had several papers retracted. Nevertheless, the whistle-blowing game remains one of swimming in shark-infested waters.

This increasingly litigious environment surrounding scientific misconduct has overwhelmingly been on the defensive side, with a far greater willingness of accused scientists to fight back in recent years. This has included scientists threatening to sue bloggers such as myself for defamation, trying to subpoena websites to gain identifying information on anonymous commenters who criticized their work, and university professors suing their institutions for wrongful dismissal or withdrawal of job offers when misconduct accusations come to light.

While such legal threats often amount to little more than chest-thumping, there can be little doubt that they have a dampening effect on the desire of whistle-blowers to speak out. Very often, legal threats from allegedly defamed individuals fall under the umbrella term "SLAPP" (Strategic Lawsuit Against Public Participation), with the goal being not to find the truth, but rather to scare the accuser into silence. Thankfully several states have anti-SLAPP statutes, and a number of lawyers committed to first amendment rights have taken active roles in defending bloggers and other online correspondents. Exemplary among these is Ken White of the popular legal blog "Pope Hat" (http://www.popehat.com/). Another key feature of such cases in the Internet age is the "Streisand Effect", named after an attempt by Barbara Streisand to prevent a website from publishing photos of her Malibu home ended up drawing far more attention to the photos than they otherwise would have received. In several recent cases, attempts by accused scientists to bring legal action have resulted in widespread reporting, often spilling over into mainstream media outlets. Key examples include Bharat Aggarwal, Rakesh Kumar, and Falzul Sarkar. Scientists who pursue such legal retribution would do well to remember the adage that scientific facts are determined empirically, not in the courts.

The other side of the legal landscape in science, i.e., when scientists sue to get to the truth, is far less populated. Hill's case serves as a biting narrative on the inadequacies of the current policing and legal systems that scientists have, in order to fight misconduct. The specific example of "Qui Tam" – in which reporters of misappropriation of government funds are entitled to a cut of any funds recovered – is touted as a readily accessible option. However, as Hill's story reveals this is far from an easy path because the bar that must be crossed to prove intentional misappropriation of funds is incredibly high. For a Qui Tam case to stick, the whistle-blower must prove that the accused knew what they were doing was wrong but did it anyway. Placing such a burden of proof on the accuser is a likely reason why there have been so few successful cases bought via this method. On this basis alone, Hill deserves accolades for having the strength and will to actually bring a Qui Tam case all the way to court.

Thus, in addition to the law, another central theme that underlies this story, it is one of perseverance. The sheer amount of mental, physical and financial effort required to bring such cases to light is often a significant deterrent to anyone considering playing the role of whistle-blower. As Hill's story illustrates, however, once the decision has been made, there is no turning back, and often the person who is already "out on a limb" must go even further still, to have any hope of bringing a case to conclusion. As readers of the popular blog "Retraction Watch", or the post-publication peer review site "PubPeer" are sadly aware, there are numerous cases in which large piles of evidence regarding alleged misconduct simply sit in public view for years or even decades, before anything is done at the government or administrative level. In many cases, the *modus operandi* on the part of journals and institutions appears to be outlasting the whistle-blowers - literally "if we ignore this for long enough it will go away". In the whistle-blowing game, staying power is an absolute must, and Hill has it in spades.

Sadly, the non-legal options available to discoverers of misconduct are no easier than the legal route. As I discovered during one of the first cases I ran across, the US Office of Research Integrity does not grant anonymity to accusers unless it is specifically requested. I wrote a detailed letter to ORI reporting on several instances of misconduct by a junior investigator, and six months later received an email from the person's supervisor thanking me for reporting! While the outcome was amicable, it is easy to imagine how things could have turned sour. When I asked ORI about this, they simply responded "you never told us you wanted to be anonymous, so we just forwarded your letter to the University". Thus, it appears even at the government regulatory level, the cards are stacked against the accuser.

On the publication end of things, the "Committee on Publication Ethics" is purportedly an organization that exists to provide *guidelines* for journals and editors, in how to deal with reports of problematic data in published papers. In my experience, COPE is little more than a trade lobbying group. It allows publishers to say "we've got this whole ethics thing covered" while continuing to obfuscate and do little to actually address issues of misconduct.

It is telling that COPE charges hefty membership fees to journals, and their guidelines specifically mention journals & publishers being *"asked to consider their continued membership"* in response to a breach of the guidelines. Yet, there is not a single example of a journal or publisher having their membership rescinded. A simple slap-on-the-wrist is all that usually happens, and the journals go back to their usual stance of least-possible-effort. Some examples I have experienced are as follows:

- Two complete six-panel figures with legends and descriptive text being reproduced in two papers in two different journals published days apart. COPE allowed both journals to publish "statements", noting that the figure was reproduced elsewhere, but not acknowledging that their guidelines on dual-simultaneous submission had been flouted. In effect, the authors double-published with zero consequences.

- A complaint to a journal about an egregious case of misconduct led to an internal investigation chaired by a scientific trainee of the paper's lead author, who was also on the journal's editorial board. The investigation found no fault. I complained to COPE, and the journal looked again and the paper was eventually retracted. No apology was received. COPE did not apply any sanctions or other punishment. The editor and the investigator at the journal still have their jobs.

- Several hundred examples of journal editors simply refusing to respond to emails. This includes not only emails from anonymous/pseudonymous persons, but emails from myself, a real person, using my institutional email address. In several cases, COPE has been CC'ed on the emails, and they too do not respond. In other cases, the person from COPE who responded, was also an editor at a different journal I had raised complaints about in the past.

The pages of Twitter, Retraction Watch, PubPeer and other sites are littered with examples of whistle-blowers being shouted down by those who do not wish to hear their message. Is it any wonder then, that the internet post-publication peer review websites (particularly those that allow anonymous commenters) have become the preferred vehicles for people to report on such matters? When all other "official" vehicles have been exhausted, there really are not many options left other than to go online and get angry.

Back to Hill's case, it should be clear that she is a pioneer in the field of science ethics. By sticking her neck out and bringing a Qui Tam case, she serves as a rare example of someone fully committed to seeing something through, rather than simply quitting due to being shouted down or counter-sued into submission, as so many others have done. She has been ostracized from her chosen career path and subjected to discrimination on a level reminiscent of the pre-civil-rights era, and yet has bounced back at every level with fresh evidence that cannot be refuted. She has remained civil, polite, and composed, and should be an example to anyone wanting a role model in how to conduct oneself in science.

Hill's case is also rare because it allows access to a side of the scientific process that few members of the public ever see. The "face" of science to most people is the popular media, with puffed-up reports claiming a cure for cancer in 5 years, or a new epilepsy drug that works in rats and will be in humans within a decade. The middle-ground is the scientific literature - unintelligible to most people, but still a polished and carefully crafted set of stories about what really went on in a laboratory. The *dark side of the moon* in science, the side never seen by the public, is the chaos of a modern laboratory... The piles of lab-books on the graduate students' desks. The critical details scribbled on post-it notes waiting to be formally documented. The Excel spreadsheets scattered across USB thumb-drives. The masses of online folders containing data and images, all with similar but ever-so-slightly different names. The millions of petri dishes sitting in freezers and incubators, their barely legible labels scrawled in sharpie marker gradually wearing off. The mass of intricate experimental details in the head of every lab scientist that simply never ever gets written down. Somehow, it is a miracle that all of this chaos can be distilled down into a reliable narrative that can be published and understood by other scientists within the context of the rest of the literature.

Is it any wonder then, that the process of going from the chaos of the lab, to the neat 30-second snippet on the evening news "health watch" section, is littered with opportunities for mistakes, and perhaps more scarily, with opportunities for perversion of information. This book provides a unique window into the path of data from lab to zeitgeist, and what happens when that path is corrupted. Perhaps the scariest message of all, between these lines, is how easy it would be for such things to happen again. This is not an isolated incident for filing away in the history books. Rather, it is a wake-up call to fix the process of science, before it is too late, and the public trust is lost.

Paul S. Brookes, Ph.D. Rochester, NY, March 2016

PREFACE

None so blind as those that will not see
Matthew Henry

Retractions of scientific papers have increased 10-fold worldwide over the past decade. Turnitin® and iThenticate®, are popular vendors of plagiarism-detection software. The latter estimates on its website[*] that there were 7 million researchers competing to publish nearly 2 million manuscripts in 31,758 scholarly journals throughout the world in 2010. They report that one leading journal published by Taylor and Francis rejected about 23% of its submissions because of plagiarism alone. Also, nearly 2% of scientists questioned in a recent study admitted to having falsified data at least once. As many as 72% of those polled had engaged in some form of questionable research practice. iThenticate® estimates that a single case of scientific misconduct costs the affected university about $525,000. In 2010, the total cost came to about $110,000,000 for investigations throughout the United States. Of even greater concern, more than 70,000 patients had been treated or otherwise participated in 859 retracted clinical studies. The iThenticate® report concludes that "time spent on research based on fraudulent work is wasted effort." I speculate that the case that I lay out in this book produced costs, real and hidden, of several million dollars.

Plagiarism software programs are valuable tools for its detection. The Office of Research Integrity (ORI) of the Department of Health and Human Services (DHHS) has downloadable software that utilizes Photoshop® for the analysis and detection of manipulated images. For statistics, however, there is no "one size fits all" solution. Programs accessible to investigators are needed that detect numbers that should be but are not random, variances, standard deviations and confidence limits that are too small or too uniform, and patterns that deviate from expectation. Several such programs were used in the pages that follow.

My story is one of the American Dream gone awry. The central character started out as a research teaching specialist -- technician

---

[*] www.ithenticate.com

-- and is now a Department Chairman in a pharmacy school in Florida. His original supervisor, a professor in my department, has supported him unflinchingly since day one. His experiments – which I question – formed the major support for a substantial government grant and its renewal and were the principal data presented in at least five of the eight papers that he co-authored while in my department – and he also contributed substantially to the other three papers. There is little doubt in my mind that the success of the oeuvre that I question has been instrumental in elevating these two individuals to distinguished positions and substantial financial support.

There were blind eyes in my department, blind eyes in my colleagues, in my university, in the US government's Office of Research Integrity, in the courts ("failure to replicate is just failure to replicate") and in the journals that refuse to publish our analyses of data that defy belief. In telling this story, I show that the system failed at every step of the way.

Being a whistle-blower is not easy. Frequently those accused are friends or colleagues. Their friends and colleagues will line up against you. Whistle-blowers are shunned or marginalized. Their motives are suspect – are they in it for the money? I think rarely. We are a breed that believe in truth – truth at all cost – and we know that we are right. To be a whistle-blower is to stick your neck out, to endanger your own position, possibly your livelihood, even your own future. Some whistle-blowers give up their careers in science. This was the case for Kathryn Milam, Ph.D. who lost her case in 1995 (*U.S. ex rel. Kathryn M. Milam v. The Regents of the University of California, et al.* Civ. No.B-90-523 (D.Md.)) and went to law school. I read of one whistle-blower who lost his home, his wife, his job yet when asked if he would do it again replied "yes".

My case is just one of a number of failures to set the record straight. In their November, 2014 newsletter, the ORI reports that in the past year they had closed 71 cases. They found misconduct in only 12 (17%). Does this mean that 59 whistle-blowers were barking up the wrong tree?

The case that woke the nation up to the fact that scientists are not the paragons that the public thought they were, known as the David Baltimore Affair, is dealt with in some detail in Chapter 16. In this well-publicized episode, post-doctoral fellow Margot

O'Toole, working in the laboratory at MIT of junior faculty member Thereza Imanishi-Kari, reported to her superiors that she believed Imanishi-Kari had fabricated data that supported a seminal paper published in the journal *Cell*. The ins and outs of the case have been dealt with in numerous newspaper articles and are the subject of two full-length books (*Science on Trial* by Judy Sarasohn, St Martin's Press, New York, 1993 and *The Baltimore Case* by Daniel J. Kevles, W.W. Norton & Co., New York, 1998). O'Toole was admired by some and vilified by others. In the intervening time since then, she worked in the pharmaceutical industry, raised a family and now has a consulting business. She is remarkably free of any resentment even though the case must certainly have shaken her up for a period of years and changed the direction of her career. The present day Office of Research Integrity (ORI) of the US Department of Health and Human Services was launched about this time and some believe was created without much backbone as a result of its poor showing in the Baltimore Case.

Recently, there was a very troubling case, won but lost by the whistle-blowers. Members of the laboratory of Elizabeth Goodwin, Ph.D., an associate professor of genetics at the University of Wisconsin, suspected that their mentor had fabricated results in two grant applications. Eventually, Dr Goodwin was found guilty in the courts, sentenced to two years of probation, fined $500 and ordered to pay $100,000 to the University. She was sanctioned by the ORI and received their usual slap on the wrist of voluntary abstention from any government contract work for 3 years or service on any Public Health Service advisory or peer review committee during that time. Goodwin appears to have recovered nicely with her own website and writing service. Her educational background is eerily similar to mine. She graduated from Smith College in 1981 (I graduated from Smith in 1950), she spent her junior year abroad, as did I, and she received her Ph.D. from Brandeis University in 1990 (my Ph.D. from Brandeis was conferred in 1964). It seems the five students who turned her in have not done as well. Their plights were cataloged in an article in *Science* in September, 2006. At that time, three were quitting school, two others were starting over. One of the three who were quitting had invested seven years in her studies, the other two, nine years between them. They complained of poor treatment by other members of the faculty who tended to side with Goodwin. Scientific misconduct wastes money, but can have hidden human collateral damage as well.

From 2000 through 2002, Robert Bauchwitz, M.D., Ph.D. assisted science journalist Gary Taubes with an article on various phases of concern in the scientific community over the work of William K. Holloman, Ph.D. and his former graduate student, Eric B. Kmiec, Ph.D. (Science. 2002 Dec 13;298(5601):2116-20). Taubes then recommended to the ORI that they contact Bauchwitz regarding additional potential research misconduct associated with Holloman and Kmiec. ORI told Bauchwitz that they had already been investigating Kmiec's "chimeraplasty" claims, which had received international scrutiny from other scientists. ORI subsequently agreed to proceed with an attempt to recover government funds through a *qui tam* suit against the defendants in which Dr. Bauchwitz was to act as relator for the government[*]. The suit was filed in 2004. The ORI was to produce a report for the Department of Justice on the science involved. In its summary ORI's Drs John Dahlberg and Alan Price stated: "Dr. Bauchwitz' complaint identifies three false claims... ORI notes that these false claims deal with only a very small portion of the much larger scope of possible misconduct issues that have been linked to Drs. Kmiec and Holloman." But for reasons still unknown, the ORI also wrote that it did not believe additional evidence would be found through the lawsuit, without providing any evidence for their "belief"[†].

Bauchwitz has claimed that the ORI's purported concern about lack of additional evidence proved to be not only inexplicable, but incorrect, as very important information was found during the limited discovery that was performed. For example, among the most clear-cut pieces of evidence obtained by subpoena from Harvard University's Microchemistry Laboratory was amino acid sequencing that the defendants had claimed was performed by that laboratory, and which was foundational to the claims that the defendants had made in scientific publications and grants. Harvard's records showed that their review had found: "These sequences are not consistent with the data we provided ... none of the sequence data we obtained agrees with the data they claimed was from our [*i.e.* Harvard's] lab ... I am confident that there is no other data." Nevertheless, Bauchwitz believes that the judge used the ORI's statements in significant part as a pretext to curtail

---

[*] Bauchwitz, R. Personal communication
[†] In my case, Dr Price, in a similar manner, stated his belief that no controls would be found, but see Table 1: there are nearly 2000 controls for colonies and 3600 for Coulter counts. Did Dr Price have a blind eye?

discovery and production of expert reports, thereby prematurely ending the case. One of the experts who reviewed the case wrote: "In every instance the evidence is strong and in many instances it is air tight. The fact that there has been no serious investigation to date shows major problems in the system." Not to be undone, Bauchwitz took fraud investigation and law courses and now devotes a significant amount of his time to helping other whistle-blowers.

In his 2002 article in *Science*, Taub states "In the 1980s, Kmiec accomplished the noteworthy feat of publishing eight articles in *Cell* based on his graduate and postdoctoral research. The central findings of the first four, however, published with his doctoral adviser William Holloman, now at Weill Medical College of Cornell University, have never been independently replicated; those of the fifth and sixth, also published with Holloman, were publicly refuted. The remaining two *Cell* papers, published as a postdoc with biologist Abraham Worcel of the University of Rochester in New York, were retracted in 1988 by Worcel, whose own lab failed to replicate the results after they were challenged by outside researchers". In my search of the web, I have failed to find any formal retractions or evidence of replication attempts.

Bauchwitz's *qui tam* case and Taub's article appear to have done little to harm Holloman and Kmiec. Holloman continues as professor of microbiology and immunology at Weill Cornell Medical College. Kmiec, whose checkered career was described in the article by Gary Taubes in *Science* in 2002, was for 4 years chairman of the chemistry department at Delaware State University in Dover but is now Director of the Gene Editing Institute of Christiana Healthcare in Wilmington, DE. The NIH has funded Kmiec's research off and on since 1999 to the tune of several million dollars, and Holloman's since 1991 for substantially more. Kmiec does not acknowledge any association with Holloman, his thesis advisor, on his Linked-In page.

ORI does not come out of this smelling like a rose. In my case as well, Dr Kay Fields, the scientist in charge of it for ORI, believed that the case should be turned back to the university for further investigation but she was overruled by her boss, Dr Price, who redacted her report so as to rule in favor of the university that there was not enough evidence for scientific misconduct. Both Fields' report and Price's revision are posted on my website (www.helenezhill.com).

Kenneth J. Jones, Ed.D., a statistician and Professor at Brandeis University, was a participant in a multi-million dollar, multi-year program project grant led by Marilyn Albert, Ph.D. who directed the studies that were carried out at the Brigham and Women's Hospital in Boston. The goal of the project was to determine whether Alzheimer's disease could be detected early in brain scans of its future victims. Ronald J. Killiany, Ph.D. measured certain brain areas seen by Magnetic Resonance Imaging in participants in the study, some of whom would go on to develop the disease. Control subjects were individuals who remained normal. Killiany did find significant differences between the controls and the Alzheimer's victims but Jones discovered that he had remeasured the targeted brain areas that earlier had shown no significant differences between the two groups. The changes in the data were not reported to the National Institute of Aging that was funding the studies and Jones instigated a case for *qui tam*. The case was filed in Boston in August, 2007 and 3 years later the judge ruled in favor of the defendants. Jones successfully appealed and the case returned to the lower court for jury trial. In July of 2013, Jones lost again and appealed again. This time, the Appeals court ruled in favor of the defendants and the case came to an end in the spring of 2015. Albert is an impressive grant swinger. Her list of successful grants from the NIH spans 23 years with jackpot sized awards. Killiany, a member of the Boston University faculty, has, himself, pulled in a couple of million dollars in government support.

There are a number of books out there that deal with fraud and misconduct in science and medicine, but few that tell the tale from the whistle-blower's point of view. To name a few: *The Whistle-blowers: exposing corruption in Government & Industry*, Basic Books, 1989 by Myron Preretz Glazer and Penina Migdal Glazer. Myron Glazer is a Professor of Sociology at Smith College. More recent books include *The Great Betrayal:Fraud in Science*, Harcourt, Inc,. 2004 by Horace Freeland Judson; *Don't Kill the Messenger: How America's valiant whistleblowers risk everything in order to speak out against waste, fraud and abuse in business and government,* Create Space Independent Publishing Platform, 2014 by Donald Ray Soeken.

Frank Wells and Michael Farthing edited the 4th edition of a series published by the Royal Society of Medicine in 2008 entitled *Fraud and Misconduct in Biomedical Research.* Chapter 15 "Handling whistle-blowers: Bane and boon" was written by C. Kristina Gunsalus, a distinguished lawyer, academician at the University of

Illinois in Urbana, ethicist and writer, and Dr Drummond Rennie, deputy editor of the New England Journal of Medicine and of the Journal of the American Medical Association, a distinguished scholar and standard bearer for poor and down-trodden whistle-blowers. In their article, they describe the plight of some whistle-blowers, as well as telling the tales of a number of alleged and established purveyors of scientific misinformation. They also provide useful guidelines and warnings for would-be whistle-blowers.

Until the scientific community figures out a way to police itself – at the local level, at the level of the granting agencies, at the level of government oversight and at the ultimate end of the line, by the journals themselves - the scientific record will remain difficult to correct. Fraudsters and charlatans will continue to survive and even to prosper.

CONTENTS

ABSTRACT

In this book, I analyze numerical data used to create graphs in eight scientific publications co-authored by (among others) a Research Teaching Specialist, Anupam Bishayee, PhD, and a laboratory director, Professor Roger W Howell, PhD. I also analyze data used to create graphs in a grant application and its Renewal awarded to Howell by the National Cancer Institute (NCI) of the National Institutes of Health (NIH). These data became available to me during the exchange of documents in Discovery relating to a *qui tam* lawsuit that I filed in October of 2003. They provided a unique opportunity to analyze virtually all of the data generated in a single laboratory over a period of approximately eight years. There were two types of data sets: counts of colonies taken in triplicate (three independent samples collected from the same original suspensions of cells) and independent cell counts taken from a Coulter particle counter, usually, but not necessarily, in triplicate, as well. The colony counts are the significant results in the graphs in the reports while the Coulter counts serve to quantify the colony counts more precisely.

I had noticed that Bishayee's data seemed to include an unusual number of triples that contained a value close to the triple's mean or equal to its exact (rounded[*]) mean. This led to the question – could the very high numbers of mean-containing triples in Bishayee's data sets have occurred merely by chance? Dr. Joel Pitt developed a probabilistic model that allows for the estimate of the probability that a given triple includes its own (rounded) mean as one of its three elements. From there, we calculate the probability that as many or more than the observed number of (rounded) mean-containing triples in a given collection of triples might have appeared merely as the result of random/chance variation. Test 1, based on Dr Pitt's model, calculates the Z-score: the difference between the actual number of (rounded) mean-containing triples, K, minus the expected number, N, divided by

---

[*] For numbers ending in 5 or more, round up (e.g. 13.5 and 13.6 round up to 14), less than 5, round down (e.g. 13.4 rounds to 13)

1

the standard deviation of N ((K-N)/σ), and the p-value associated with that Z-score (p≥K).

Test 2 uses the well-known Chi squared test to check the hypothesis that the rightmost terminal digits in given sets of data were generated uniformly. Higher Chi squared values correspond to less uniform sets. The corresponding p-value is the probability that the set of digits drawn from a uniform distribution is as non-uniform as the actual set of terminal digits. Test 3 calculates the probability that the two rightmost terminal digits in given sets of Coulter data will be equal, given the expectation of 10% for that equality.

There were 5187 Coulter counts from 174 experiments in Bishayee's notebooks and 2987 Coulter counts from 103 experiments in the notebooks of eight others in the Radiation Research Lab using the same Coulter counter. There were also 687 Coulter counts in 23 experiments provided by two outside laboratories. There were 1362 triplicate counts of colonies in 128 experiments reported by Bishayee, 586 triplicate colony counts in 59 experiments conducted by nine other investigators in the same Radiation Research Lab, and 50 triplicate colony counts from one experiment provided by an outside laboratory.

By test 1, the probability that the averages in Bishayee's colony triples are equal to, or greater than expected is not significantly different from 0 and the probability that the averages in his Coulter triples are equal to, or greater than expected is 2.40×10^{-14}. For all the other investigators, the probabilities are 0.792 and 0.999 respectively, i.e. are consistent with expectation. By test 2, the probability that Bishayee's Coulter terminal digits are uniform is not significantly different from 0 and for his colony terminal digits, that probability is 2.33×10^{-38}. For all the others, the probabilities are 0.104 and 0.964, respectively, i.e. are consistent with uniform. By test 3, the two terminal digits of Coulter counts should be equal 10% of the time. 12.4% of Bishayee's Coulter counts have terminal doubles, probability 1.08×10^{-8}, and for all other investigators, 9.8% of Coulter counts have terminal doubles, probability 0.693.

Bishayee started the first experiment suggesting deviations from expected of both Coulter and colony counts on December 4, 1997, approximately two months after he began working in the Lab.

Working with the several thousand PDF files of scans from the laboratory notebooks available to me during the discovery period of the *qui tam* law suit, I determined which experiments were used to draw the graphs in the Figures of the eight papers co-authored by Howell and Bishayee and in the grant and Renewal applications. I tabulate my calculations in this book. Further, I argue that the survival and bystander results presented in two of the papers are not plausible under the conditions that prevailed in the experiments. In fact, Howell himself and a post-doctoral fellow were unable to replicate them. These arguments and replication attempts appear in our publication, Hill and Pitt, *Publications* 2: 71-82. I also present figures from Bishayee's publications since leaving the New Jersey Medical School that raise questions regarding the possibility that the photographs of gels represented therein may have been rearranged.

Dr John Carlisle is a scientist well known for his statistical analyses of numerical data reported in an anaesthesiology journal that resulted in the retraction of some 183 reports. He has added his expertise to the study of the data from the Radiation Research Lab. He concludes that Bishayee's (investigator O's) results are not reliable and that reports based on them should be retracted.

Useful programs exist to deal with plagiarism and image manipulation (cf the ORI website). In writing this book, I hope to convince the scientific community of the need to apply statistical methods to the analysis of all raw numerical data that underlie graphs and charts in reports and grant applications. The time has come for statistical analysis to take its place in routine data analysis to further reduce opportunities for scientific misconduct. It is important to remember that numbers lie behind every graph.

1. INTRODUCTION

Yesterday is gone. Tomorrow has yet to come. We have only today. Let us begin.

Mother Teresa

In 1999, I, a Professor of Radiology at the NJ Medical School in Newark, observed what I believed was questionable behavior on the part of a Research Teaching Specialist, Anupam Bishayee, Ph.D., who worked alongside me. In 2001, a second worker in the Lab, a post-doctoral Fellow, Marek Lenarczyk, Ph.D., who also worked beside Bishayee, reported to me additional questionable behavior on the part of Bishayee. I documented my observations and later reported them to the University Campus Committee on Research Integrity (CCRI). The CCRI ruled that there was insufficient evidence of research misconduct. I disagreed and subsequently reported my findings to the Office of Research Integrity (ORI) of the Department of Health and Human Services (DHHS). This, too, proved futile as the ORI decided to support the University. However, they had uncovered suspicious numerical evidence using a technique developed by a statistician, James E. Mosimann, who had previously worked for the ORI. I used this method to expose additional questionable numerical evidence in Bishayee's experimental data. I then requested a new investigation by the CCRI, following the suggestion of the investigators at the ORI. This second hearing by the CCRI again proved futile because the second CCRI ignored the new data.

In October, 2003, frustrated by my inability to convince these bodies of scientific misconduct, I turned to the courts at the suggestion of one of the ORI investigators, hoping to obtain a ruling that false information had been used in an application for a government grant. This type of lawsuit is known as a *qui tam*. In such a suit, a whistle-blower (Relator) charges on behalf of the government that there has been a violation of the False Claims Act on the part of the defendants. After 3½ years of investigations, the US Attorney decided not to take the case and turned it over to me for prosecution. During the period known as Discovery (a legal process during which the various parties exchange information) a large number of Portable Document Format (PDF) files were turned over to me. These consisted of scans of most, if not all, of the Lab notebooks during an eight year period that spanned

Bishayee's four years in the Lab. It is the experiments contained in these files that form the body of the studies analyzed in this book.

The Discovery materials included on the order of 30,000 PDF files many of which were irrelevant and immaterial. Nevertheless, I was able to distill out over 400 experiments, roughly 60% of which had been performed by Bishayee. Nine other workers performed the other 40% in the same Lab using the same or similar techniques. Also, data obtained using similar methods were sent to me from three outside laboratories. It is customary in such lawsuits to procure the testimony of expert witnesses. I employed the services of two experts: Joel H Pitt, Ph.D., a statistician, and Michael Robbins, Ph.D., a radiation biologist. It is in this manner that Dr. Pitt and I became collaborators on research publications. The testimony of Dr. Robbins was also essential in confirming the radiation biology principles that I discuss in a later chapter and that form the substance of the analysis in our publication (Hill and Pitt, *Publications* 2: 71-82). Unfortunately, Dr. Robbins died in November 2012.

On October 18, 2010, the Hon. Judge Dennis Cavanagh of the United States District Court in the District of New Jersey ruled in favor of the defendants that there had been no violation of the False Claims Act. In his opinion, Howell was exonerated as he had not known that the government had been defrauded at the moment that he submitted his grant application to the NIH in 1999. However, he was almost sure to know later on and even, in fact, before he presented an application for renewal of the grant in 2005. Although, in the eyes of the USPHS, a renewal has the same status as a new grant application, the judge did not think so. The judge further ruled that Bishayee was not material to the case, even though he had performed most of the experiments that were cited as crucial preliminary results in the grant application. The judge totally disregarded statistical evidence that was presented by Dr. Pitt. Howell and post-doctoral fellow Lenarczyk had attempted to replicate certain of Bishayee's experiments 22 times and failed (*vide ultra:* Chapter 8). The judge in his wisdom stated that failure to replicate is simply failure to replicate. He thereby entirely disregarded one of the most central tenets of the scientific method: that replication is the cornerstone for acceptance of scientific validity. On December 12, 2012, three judges of the

United States Court of Appeals for the Third District confirmed and supported Judge Cavanaugh's ruling. Earlier, Judge Dolores Sloviter, one of the three judges, had introduced the oral arguments by saying "We are just judges... I never had a science course in my life".

Once these decisions had come down, I submitted new material, gleaned from Discovery, and that I present in the chapters that follow, to a third CCRI. I also made a second attempt to make a presentation to the ORI. It appears that this third seating of the CCRI was a monkey trial, and it failed. I never received any official report. The ORI, on the other hand, refused even to review the new material that was presented to them, stating incorrectly that they had already reviewed it.

Regardless of the fact that three attempts failed to convince the CCRI, two attempts failed to convince the ORI that scientific misconduct had occurred, and that Judge Cavanagh supported by the Court of Appeals ruled that there was no violation of the False Claims Act, I believe that they are wrong. It is one purpose of this book to so demonstrate.

Further, it is the goal of this book to show the power of statistics at revealing anomalous, potentially falsified data. It is an additional purpose to make evident that institutions of higher learning are not necessarily objective when it comes to investigating their academic faculty and scientific staff, especially when large amounts of money are involved. The grants affected in reports that I analyze here amounted to nearly 2½ million dollars. I stress the need for impartial scientific courts to judge scientists and to rule on scientific misconduct.

In this case, the system failed at the level of the laboratory where the experiments were performed, at the level of the University and its scientific review, at the level of the government – the ORI standing for the funding agencies of the National Institutes of Health -- at the level of the judiciary, and at the level of journal publishers who fear retribution in the form of lawsuits. The system for dealing with scientific misconduct needs to change.

2. THE DATA SETS

Cherish those who seek the truth but beware of those who find it

Voltaire

There are two categories of data in the experiments that Dr. Pitt and I analyzed: Coulter counts and colony counts. The Coulter counter is an instrument that counts particles, in this case, single mammalian tissue culture cells in liquid suspension. A specific volume is pulled by a vacuum through a tiny orifice, thereby producing an electrical signal with the passage of each cell. The count for each given volume, which is to say for each experimental sample, is recorded on a light-emitting diode (LED) screen. Investigators in the Radiation Research Lab copied the screen number to a table that was included in the results for each experiment. The LED record is similar to the gallon counter on a gas pump. Large numbers of cells pass through the orifice hence the terminal – rightmost - digit of the count is insignificant and equally probable to be any one of the ten integers 0, 1, 2, etc. Furthermore, where the numbers of digits are sufficiently large – in the hundreds or thousands -- the terminal digit will be equal to the second rightmost digit about 10% of the time.

The colony results in most experiments were usually obtained as follows: tissue culture cells from suspensions were counted, apportioned into culture tubes and incubated overnight with radioisotopes. After (usually) a twelve-hour incubation, the investigator harvested and washed the cells by centrifugation to remove unincorporated radioactivity. S/he transferred the cells to new tubes (Helena tubes, tall, narrow plastic centrifuge tubes purchased from the Helena Plastics Company) to be incubated at low temperature for three days. This long incubation in the cold allows any incorporated radioisotopes to decay in the absence of any cell division (100% experiments). In some experiments, washed cells previously exposed to radioactivity were mixed with naïve cells for the low-temperature incubation (50% and 10% experiments: in the former, 50% of the cells in the Helena tubes are radioactive; in the latter, 10% in the cells are radioactive). The cells were harvested after the three days of cold incubation, suspended in culture medium, and then small portions (aliquots) were transferred in triplicate to vials for Coulter counting. A separate aliquot was serially diluted and equal volumes were distributed into three independent tissue culture dishes containing growth medium. The individual cells adhere to the bottom surfaces of the culture dishes. The dishes are incubated for about one week at 37° C (about 98.6° F). Cells that have survived the radiation treatment replicate to form colonies. Figure 1, taken from the literature, shows a photograph of a 60 mm diameter tissue culture dish containing colonies of mammalian cells.[1]

The following radionuclides were used in the various experiments that follow: tritiated water, ^3H_2O; tritiated thymidine, ^3H-thymidine or ^3HTdR; ^{131}Iodo-uridine or ^{131}IdU; ^{125}Iodo-uridine or ^{125}IdU; ^{210}Polonium citrate or ^{210}Po; $^{117m}Sn(4+)$diethyltriaminepentaacetic acid (tin DTPA) and external beam gamma ray emitting ^{137}Cesium (^{137}Cs). In any one experiment, all the Coulter counts for all the samples are expected to be roughly the same. Each sample starts out with about the same number of cells. All the samples are incubated in the cold for three days which should inhibit cell division, so their numbers are not expected to change. The radioactivity only affects the replicative ability of the exposed cells and that effect should not be expressed until after the cells are plated singly for colonies and incubated at 37° C to allow them to replicate.

There are six data sets: 5187 Coulter and 4086 colony counts are from Bishayee's experiments. 2987 Coulter and 1758 colony counts are from experiments by others in the Radiation Research Lab. 687 Coulter counts are from two outside laboratories, and 150 colony counts are from a third outside laboratory.

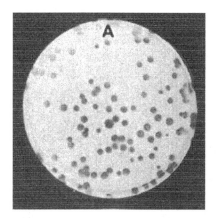

Figure 1. A 60mm tissue culture dish containing colonies of V79 Chinese hamster cells that have been fixed and stained. The colonies are counted by inverting the dish and marking the bottom of the dish over each colony as it is counted. © Permission of the Genetics Society of America. Different individuals might have slightly different counts depending on what they might consider distinct colonies.

3. STATISTICAL TESTS

I generally believe people should be data savvy, and we should teach statistics in high school...and the reason is the world today really revolves around analytics...So the ability to think data, the ability to speak data, to understand the power of data, I think every citizen on this planet should understand, because it's so powerful
        Sebastian Thrun

The publications by Pitt and Hill describe in greater detail the three tests applied in the discussions that follow.[2]

Test 1: Each colony and Coulter count was acquired independently. The rounded average of the triples in Bishayee's data frequently appeared as one of the triples, especially in the colony counts. It seemed unlikely that this phenomenon would occur by chance. Dr Pitt proposed a model that calculates the probability of getting as many or more than the actual numbers of means or averages in a given set of triples.[2] Figure 2 is a scan from a notebook page of colony counts in an experiment performed by Bishayee. The highlighted rounded average appears as one of the triplicate counts in nine of the ten samples.

Expt #: 2   Date: 04/22/99

Colony Counts and Survival Fraction

MidRatio	Tube dilution	Colony 1	Colony 2	Colony 3	Avg Colony (/2)	SF
0.63	1.2	130	144	142	140.33	---
0.50	2.2	131	137	143	137.0	0.9762
0.53	3.2	123	135	138	130.66	0.9311
0.50	4.2	128	134	140	134	0.9548
0.45	5.2	125	131	136	130.33	0.9287
0.50	6.3	115	126	137	126	0.089
0.43	7.2	17	20.33	24	20.33	0.1484
0.50	8.2	29	35	41	35	0.2678
0.50	9.2	62	70	54	62	0.4626
0.47	10.2	70.33	79	62	70.33	0.5396

Figure 2. A scan from Bishayee's notebook showing colony count triples, nine out of 10 of which contain the highlighted (rounded) average. The probability for such occurrence according to the Pitt model is 4.23×10^{-9} (only 1.5 ± 1.1 averages are expected by the Pitt model). The left-hand column is the mid-ratio for each triple.

The mid-ratio calculation made on each triple: the middle value minus the lowest value is divided by the highest value minus the lowest value. When the mid-value is close to the mean, the quotient, i.e., the mid-ratio, will be close to 0.5. The left-hand column in Figure 2 shows the mid-ratios for the triples in each row of Figure 2. The distribution of mid-ratios provides a useful graphic method of visualizing the excess of average or near average values in a series of triples, see below.

Test 2: Mosimann *et al.*[3] recommend a method for recognizing aberrant, and potentially fabricated, numbers. They hypothesized that the least significant digits of data generated by such instruments as the scintillation counter, which records radioactive decay - a series of random events - will be randomly or uniformly distributed. They further demonstrated that many individuals are unable to invent numbers in a random fashion. This second test uses the chi-square test for independence to determine the probability that the terminal digits of arrays of Coulter and colony counts are random or uniform. The comparison arrays were ten equal numbers totaling the same as the test arrays. Since the colonies were hand-counted, the terminal digits could well be influenced by the experimenter either consciously or unconsciously. Therefore, test 2 is less robust when applied to colony counts, in contrast to the Coulter counts that come (allegedly) from a machine.

Test 3: it is reasonable to expect that in randomly generated numbers, the next to rightmost digits should be equal to the terminal digits 10% of the time. In this test, the frequency of terminal duplicates in the Coulter counts, which are all three or more digits in length is calculated, and their binomial probability is determined.

Test 1 is most *á propos* for colony data, and tests 2 and 3 are most *á propos* for Coulter data. Individual unconscious idiosyncrasies and numerical preferences could influence colony terminal digit recording (Tests 2 and 3) without actually indicating any duplicity. On the other hand, Coulter terminal digit records depend entirely on the machine and should not be subject to any influence by the operator. The average of the three colony counts is bound to appear in the triples from time to time (Test 1), but its *frequent* appearance causes concern. In most of the Tables that follow, I show the results mainly of Test 1 for colony counts and the results mainly of Test 2 for Coulter counts, unless Test 1 for Coulters and Test 2 for colonies are remarkable. In some of our analyses, the Test 3 results were not remarkable, and I only include them in Tables where they appear to be significant. In the Tables that follow, grey-scale backgrounds denote entries relevant for colony counts and Coulter counts. Test 1 results are lightest in color, Test 2 results are intermediate, and Test 3 are darkest. P-values less than 0.05 are in bold. In general, statisticians consider p-values less than 0.05 to be *significant* and less than 0.001 are *highly significant*. Many of Bishayee's p-values are far less than 0.001.

I copied data from PDF files sent to me by the defendants during the Discovery phase of the *qui tam* lawsuit. Those data are arranged in my original spreadsheets in rows of triples, although some rows may contain missing values. Rows with missing values are not suitable for analysis by Test 1, but Tests 2 and 3 analyze entries individually. Pitt has developed a spreadsheet known as The Analyzer© that refers to a second (designated) spreadsheet containing rows of data. The tests are applied to designated rows in the selected sheet. PDF files containing all the raw data and Excel files containing all the data used by the Analyzer© are available to the public on the website Open Science Framework (https://osf.io). All data in the spreadsheets at the OSF website are listed by Bates numbers allowing them to be located (and verified) in the accompanying PDF files.

In the Tables that follow, the Analyzer© calculated the results using the appropriate Excel files listed on the OSF website.

4. CONTROLS

There is, however, no genius so gifted as not to need control and verification

John Tyndall

Nine other members of the Radiation Research Lab than Bishayee used the same Coulter counter and counted colonies in the same manner. Their Coulter and colony counts serve as controls, as does data sent from the three outside laboratories. Table 1 shows the analysis of these control data based on all three tests and contrasts them with the analysis of all of Bishayee's data using those tests[*]. Probabilities less than 10^{-40} (0.000...01, 39 zeros after the decimal point) are too small to estimate precisely. However, they are shown here as calculated by the Analyzer© to emphasize the extreme improbability of some results.

It is evident from the results of all three tests in Table 1 that Bishayee's results are not likely to be due to randomness or chance alone, in contrast to the results of all the others. Bishayee's colony $P(\geq K)$ and the Coulter Terminal Digit Chi Square p are essentially 0. I have left the probability calculations from the Excel Spread Sheet to emphasize their infinitesimal nature. The Control results in Table 1 (Lab, Outside1,-2,-3) for both colonies and Coulters are entirely consistent with the expectations of randomness or chance for all three of the tests.

---

[*] Z-scores or Z-values are well-known to students of statistics in many different fields of study. Pitt's model calculates the expected number of means (N) in a given set of data triples and the corresponding standard deviation. The z-score is the number of standard deviations the actual number of averages (K) is above (or below for a negative score) the mean, the p is its associated probability ($p \geq K$).

Colonies

	# Exps	Total Data	# Triples /Total	K=# w Mean	N=# Exp'd	SD	Z-Value	P≥K	Term. Digits Chi Sq p
Lab	62	1834	578/597	109	112.3	9.4	-0.4	0.7	1.0
Outside1	1	150	49/50	3	7.9	2.6	-2.1	1.0	0.2
Bishayee	128	4085	1343/1361	690	220.4	13.4	35	2.6×10^{-265}	2.3×10^{-38}

Table 1 Colonies: columns 4-9, light grey, pertain to Test 1, darker grey columns 3 and 10 to Test 2. Re: # Triples: upper value is the number of qualifying triples (complete triples with a gap (high count – low count) $\geq$ 2), lower value is the total number of complete triples. K, number of rounded mean-containing triples; N, number expected based on the Pitt model[2]; SD is standard deviation of N; Z-score is calculated using the Pitt model; P≥K Probability of as many or more than K triples based on the Pitt model. Darker grey: Chi-squared probability for terminal digit uniform distribution.

Coulters

	# Exps	Total Data	# Triples	K=# w Mean	N=# Exp'd	SD	Z-Value	P≥K	Term Digits Chi Sq p	% Term. Dbls	P(dbls)
Lab	103	2942	929/929	36	48.8	6.8	-2.0	1.0	0.07	9.9	0.6
Outside2	11	315	97/97	0	5.4	2.3	-2.6	1.0	0.4	10.2	0.5
Outside3	17	360	120/120	1	4.4	2.1	-1.9	1.0	0.8	8.3	0.9
Bishayee	174	5185	1726/1727	176	99.9	9.7	7.8	2.4×10^{-14}	7.1×10^{-95}	12.4	1.0×10^{-8}

Table 1. **Coulters:** Light grey columns 4-9 pertain to Test 1, darker grey columns 3 and 10 to Test 2 and darkest grey columns, 11 and 12 to Test 3: percent and probability of terminal doubles.

5. BISHAYEE'S EXPERIMENTS

Choice not chance determines your destiny

Aristotle

Bishayee began working in the Radiation Research Laboratory in October 1997 and ended in July of 2001. Figure 3 shows Test 1 and Test 2 probabilities for experiments performed in the laboratory over the period of 1/1/1995 to 1/1/2003. Bishayee conducted experiments that involved six different incorporated radioisotopes and a ^{137}Cs external beam irradiator. In Figure 3A, Bishayee's probabilities ($P \geq K$) for the mean appearance in colony triples in 128 experiments fall below p=0.05 for 102, below 0.01 for 89 and below 0.001 for 69 experiments. Only 2 of the 52 experiments of others in the Lab fall below 0.05, exactly what would be expected. Bishayee performed the first experiment to fall below probability of 0.05 in December 1997, scarcely two months after his arrival in the Lab. Figure 3B shows the chi-squared probabilities for the Coulter terminal digit counts made in the Lab during the same period. For 45 of these experiments, the hypothesis that the terminal digits of these counts were drawn uniformly would be rejected at the 0.01 level, all 45 were performed by Bishayee. The many experiments in which Bishayee's distributions gave a probability greater than 0.01 are an indication that the Coulter counter was not malfunctioning.

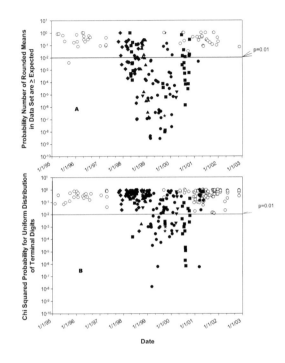

Figure 3. Bishayee's experiments are shown as filled symbols and those of others in the Lab as open symbols. **3A**. Colony count probabilities based on test 1. Values below the 0.01 line are all Bishayee's with one exception. **3B**. Chi-squared probabilities for uniform distribution of rightmost Coulter terminal digits based on Test 2. Only Bishayee's Coulter results fall below the 0.01 line. ^{131}IdU: diamonds; ^{125}IdU: squares; $^{3}H_2O$: crosses; ^{3}H-thymidine: black circles; ^{117m}Sn-DTPA: inverted triangles; ^{210}Po-citrate: triangles; ^{137}Cs external beam: stars; open circles: controls: other investigators.

Figure 4 shows the mid-ratios for the colony counts of the various isotopes Bishayee used in his experiments. 4A is a profile of control (all others in the Lab) triples. Contrast that to B – H, profiles of all the various isotopes with which Bishayee worked during his four years in the Lab. More than half of Bishayee's triples for all the isotopes occur in the distribution range of 0.4-0.6. The p ($\geq$K) for the means appearing in the triples of various isotopes are recorded in the Figure legend. Four of the seven are less than 10^{-40}, expressed as 0.

Mid-Ratio (mid-lo)/hi-lo)

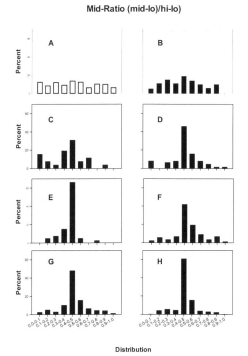

Distribution

Figure 4. Distributions of the mid-ratios, broken down by isotope, P$\geq$K probabilities in parentheses – a 0 indicates too small (P$\geq$K< 10^{-40}) to estimate. **A.** 468 triples, Controls – all other investigators in the Lab (0.93); **B.** 185 triples, ^{131}IdU experiments (3.24x10^{-8}); **C.** 36 triples, external beam ^{137}Cs experiments (4.40x10^{-4}); **D.** 89 triples, ^{3}H$_2$O experiments (0); **E.** 50 triples, ^{117m}Sn-DTPA experiments (2.17x10^{-12}); **F.** 140 triples, ^{210}Po-citrate experiments (0); **G.** 388 triples, ^{125}IdU experiments (0); **H.** 456 triples, ^{3}Hthymidne experiments (0).

Most of the relevant experiments analyzed here are designed to measure cell (colony) survivals as a function of dose. The mean value of each triple is a measure of survival for each particular treatment or dose. Survival curves are constructed by using a line to fit the survival points best. An investigator wishing to guide the survival results as they will appear on a graph could calculate the desired mean colony number for each dose and choose values equidistant on either side for the error bars. Mid-ratios that cluster in the 0.4 – 0.6 range reflect this tendency.

Table 2 represents the terminal digit distributions for Coulter and colony counts of the various investigators in this study. Bishayee's Coulter terminal distributions contrast to others in the Radiation Research Lab and the two outside laboratories and his colony distributions contrast to others in the Radiation Research lab and a third outside laboratory. Colony counts reflect an element of individual decision making (see Figure 1). Nevertheless, the Control colony terminal digits are consistent with uniformity while those of Bishayee are not. The Table also shows the digit distributions of terminal doubles. Here, again, Bishayee's are non-random while those of the Controls (Others in the Radiation Research Lab) are consistent with random.

In their articles, Mosimann et al.[3] remark on the inability when asked of many individuals to generate strings of random numbers. It seems that some underlying psychological prejudices or beliefs may guide choices of digits (too many of some, too few of others). In Table 2, only Bishayee's p-values are less than 0.05, in fact much less than 0.05. His distributions show a paucity of 4's for both Coulter and colonies.

		Digit											Chi-sq	P-value
Type	Investigator	0	1	2	3	4	5	6	7	8	9	Total	Chi-sq	P-value
Coulter	Bishayee 174 experiments	475	613	736	416	335	732	363	425	372	718	5185	466.9	7×10^{-95}
Coulter	Others 103 experiments	261	311	295	259	318	290	298	283	331	296	2942	16.0	0.067
Coulter	Outside lab 11 experiments	28	34	29	24	27	36	44	33	26	33	314	9.9	0.40
Coulter	Outside lab 17 experiments	34	38	45	35	32	42	31	35	35	33	360	4.9	0.84
Colonies	Bishayee 128 experiments	564	324	463	313	290	478	336	408	383	526	4085	200.5	2.3×10^{-38}
Colonies	Others 62 experiments	191	181	195	179	184	175	178	185	185	181	1834	1.8	0.99
Colonies	Outside lab 1 experiment	21	9	15	16	19	19	9	19	11	12	150	12.1	0.21
Doubles	Bishayee 174 experiments	27	124	88	58	43	81	68	38	52	57	636	113.1	3.4×10^{-20}
Doubles	Others 103 experiments	18	29	34	21	25	31	29	29	37	25	278	10.6	0.30

Table 2. Terminal digit distributions of Coulter and colony entries of various individuals in the study. Values in each row were compared to appropriately corresponding uniform distributions. For example, Bishayee's Coulter digits were compared to 518.5 for each of the ten integers.

Figure 5 is a graphic representation of the Coulter and colony terminal digit distributions recorded in Table 2 for members of the

Radiation Research Lab. Note the similarity of Bishayee's colony and Coulter distribution patterns. There is an abundance of digits 2, 5, and 9 in both sets, and a paucity of 4's in both sets.

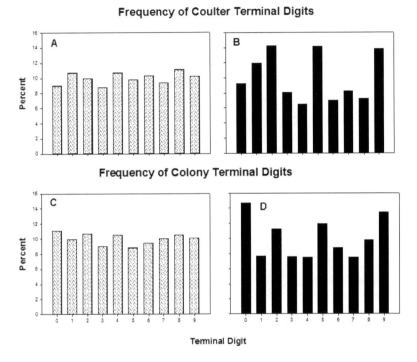

Figure 5. Terminal Digit Distributions of Coulter and Colony counts in the Radiation Research Lab. **A.** Coulters, Other investigators; **B.** Coulters, Bishayee. **C.** Colonies, Other Investigators; **D.** Colonies, Bishayee.

6. THE GRANT APPLICATION AND ITS RENEWAL

Three things cannot be long hidden: the sun, the moon and the truth   Buddha

R01-CA083838: EFFECTS OF NONUNIFORM DISTRIBUTIONS OF RADIOACTIVITY

Howell submitted the grant application to the NIH on October 21, 1999. The Radiation Study Section reviewed it. Funding started July 1, 2001, and continued until June 30, 2006. The total payout was $1,222,268. This will be referred to as grant #1 in discussions that follow. The Radiation Therapeutics and Biology Study Section reviewed the renewal application, referred to as the Renewal in discussions that follow. Funding for the Renewal ran from July 2006, through May 2011, for a total payout of $978,939. In all, the Principal Investigator, Howell, and the University received $2,201,207 for these studies.

There are 12 figures in the funded application for grant #1. I compared survival results with experiments found in the Discovery materials, and I identified and analyzed background numerical data for Figures 1A and B, 2, 3, 4, 6, 7, 11 and 12. Figures 5, 8 and 9 depict Fluorescence Activated Cell Sorter (FACS) profiles, 10 is a diagram and 12 presents the same data as Figure 2 but uses different units for the abscissa. At the time of submission of the Renewal, Bishayee had been gone from the Radiation Research Lab for several years. I was only able to identify one figure (C1) that contained data generated by him.

Table 3 depicts the statistical analysis of the data found in 8 Figures in grant #1 and the Renewal. Bishayee was the investigator for all of the matched experiments. Regarding Figure C1 of the Renewal, Howell states that both sets of experiments had been published. The upper graph in Renewal Figure C1 depicts three survival curves for tritiated thymidine. The 10% curve (squares) was taken from Figure 2B of Bishayee, Hill *et al*. (2001)[4] (paper #7 in the list below). The 50% curve (triangles) is taken from Figure 2A-circles, from that same paper. The 100% curve (circles) was taken from Figure 3 of the Bishayee, Rao and Howell paper (1999)[5] (paper #6 in the list below). Each plot from the upper Renewal Figure C1 is analyzed separately in my Table 3 that follows below as each came from a different source. The lower graph in Figure C1 of the Renewal represents three survival curves for ^{125}IdU published as Figure 2 in the *Micron* paper (paper #8 in the list below, *q.v.*). Table 3 shows only the accumulated results of those three individual experiments.

In Table 3-Colonies, the only probabilities greater than 0.05 are for Figures 1B and 11 of the grant #1 application. As there are only ten triples in each of these experiments, the relatively high probability for p$\geq$K may be due to small sample size. For 16 of the 18 graphs analyzed in grant #1 application and the Renewal, the p$\geq$K probabilities are all less than 0.05, in fact, 13 probabilities are less than 10^{-4}. Ten of the Coulter probabilities for uniformity of the terminal digits fall below 0.02, and 6 fall below 10^{-3}. In the aggregate, there were 1322 Coulter counts, 199 (15.1%) of which contained duplicate terminal digits, 132 (10%) were expected. The probability of 199 is 5.48×10^{-9} (data not shown).

Had the Study Sections that reviewed these applications been aware of these probabilities, would they have ranked grant #1 and Renewal in the fundable range? The judge in the *qui tam* case did not believe that knowledge of these probabilities would have made any difference as regards to the awarding of the grant. I disagree.

Howell has obtained additional funding from the USPHS following his above support from the National Cancer Institute. From September 1, 2007 through 28 February, 2011, he was funded by the National Institute for Allergy and Infectious Diseases for a project entitled PROTECTION AGAINST RADIATION-INDUCED DAMAGE TO INTESTINAL NUTRIENT TRANSPORT for a total funding of $1,057,387. In that application, he cites all three of the group 3 papers (below) as preliminary support for his proposal, as well as listing them in his Biographical Sketch. This grant will be referred to as Grant #2 in the ensuing discussions. More recently, he, along with Edouard Azzam, have been funded for three years for a project from the National Cancer Institute entitled RADIATION INDUCED BYSTANDER EFFECTS IN RADIUM-223 THERAPY. The total first year funding is $421,612. Both papers in the Journal of Nuclear Medicine (papers 4 and 5 below) are cited in the list of references in that application. Howell also lists those two papers along with paper number one (below) in his Biographical Sketch that accompanies that application. This grant will be referred to as Grant #3 in the ensuing discussions. Copies of all grant applications were obtained through requests from FOIA.

Figure	Type	Radio-nuclide	Symbol	# Exps	Colonies			SD	Z-Value	P≥K
					Qual triples/Total	#w Mean	#Exp			
1A	100%	^{210}Po	Closed Sq	2	20/20	8	3.4	1.7	2.5	**0.01**
1A	10%	^{210}Po	Open Sq	2	20/20	15	2.9	1.6	7.4	**1.8x10^{-12}**
1B	10%	^{131}IdU	Open Cir	1	10/10	2	1.3	1.1	0.2	0.4
2	100%	^{3}HdThd	Triangle	2	20/20	12	3.1	1.6	5.2	**1.0x10^{-6}**
2	50%	^{3}HdThd	Circle	2	19/19	14	3.0	1.6	6.7	**2.3x10^{-10}**
2	10%	^{3}HdThd	Square	2	20/20	13	3.0	1.6	6.0	**2x10^{-8}**
3	Lindane Conc	^{3}HdThd	Circle Square Triangle	3	15/15	15	2.4	1.4	8.6	**2.8x10^{-16}**
4	-	^{3}HdThd	Triangle	2	19/19	14	3.0	1.6	6.7	**2.3x10^{-10}**
4	+DMSO	^{3}HdThd	Circle	2	20/20	12	2.9	1.6	5.5	**2.9x10^{-7}**
4	+Lindane	^{3}HdThd	Diamond	2	20/20	17	2.9	1.6	8.7	**1.0x10^{-16}**
4	+Lin+ DMSO	^{3}HdThd	Square	2	20/20	17	3.1	1.6	8.3	**2.0x10^{-15}**
6	Acute & Chronic	^{137}Cs	Diamond	2	16/16	7	2.9	1.5	2.3	**0.02**
7	Clusters /susp	^{137}Cs	Circle Diamond	1	10/10	7	1.4	1.1	4.6	**2.6x10^{-5}**
11	+/- DMSO	^{125}IdU	Circle	1	10/10	2	1.5	1.1	0.0	0.4
C1 Upper	10%	^{3}HdThd	Square	2	20/20	13	3.0	1.6	6.0	**2x10^{-8}**
C1 Upper	50%	^{3}HdThd	Triangle	3	29/29	19	4.3	1.9	7.5	**1.1x10^{-12}**
C1 Upper	100%	^{3}HdThd	Circle	2	20/20	12	3.1	1.6	5.2	**1.0x10^{-6}**
C1 Lower	10% 50% 100%	^{125}IdU	Circle Square Triangle	3/6/6	133/135	76	24.5	4.3	11.7	**4.0x10^{-30}**

Table 3 Colonies

Figure	Type	Radio-nuclide	Symbol	# Exps	# Term Digits	Term Dig Chi Sq P
					Coulter Counts	
1A	100%	^{210}Po	Closed Sq	2	60	0.14
1A	10%	^{210}Po	Open Sq	2	60	0.35
1B	10%	^{131}IdU	Open Cir	1	30	0.12
2	100%	^{3}HdThd	Triangle	2	60	0.28
2	50%	^{3}HdThd	Circle	2	60	1.3×10^{-2}
2	10%	^{3}HdThd	Square	2	60	1.7×10^{-7}
3	Lindane Conc	^{3}HdThd	Circle Square Triangle	3	45	0.10
4	-	^{3}HdThd	Triangle	2	60	1.3×10^{-2}
4	+DMSO	^{3}HdThd	Circle	2	60	4.5×10^{-8}
4	+Lindane	^{3}HdThd	Diamond	2	60	1.5×10^{-4}
4	+Lin+DMSO	^{3}HdThd	Square	2	54	1.1×10^{-2}
6	Acute & Chronic	^{137}Cs	Diamond	2	48	0.47
7	Clusters susp	^{137}Cs	Circle Diamond	1	20	7.4×10^{-13}
11	+/- DMSO	^{125}IdU	Circle	1	30	0.47
C1 Upper	10%	^{3}HdThd	Square	2	60	1.7×10^{-7}
C1 Upper	50%	^{3}HdThd	Triangle	3	90	6.5×10^{-3}
C1 Upper	100%	^{3}HdThd	Circle	2	60	0.28
C1 Lower	10% 50% 100%	^{125}IdU	Circle Square Triangle	3/6/6	405	1.8×10^{-43}

Table 3 Coulters

Table 3: Analysis of Data from Graphs in Grant Application and Renewal. The Table shows Test 1 results for colony counts (light grey) and Test 2 results for Coulter counts (darker grey). Column 1 in the Table lists the figures in the grant (numerals) and Renewal (C1 upper and lower). Columns 2 – 5 are as stated in the headers. In column 6 colonies, qualifying triples were those for which the differences between the highest and lowest count was ≥ 2 ("numerator") over the total number of triples ("denominator"). For further explanation, see Table 1.

7. THE PUBLICATIONS

The eyes are useless when the mind is blind
Evan Carmichael

Bishayee co-authored eight papers with Howell while he worked in the Lab. I matched the graphs in the figures with results in the Discovery PDF documents. Usually, the number of experiments found corresponded to the number cited in the figure legends of the papers. When they did not, I determined which ones gave the most appropriate fit. The analyses that follow rely on the best possible matching of experiments in the Discovery material with the plots shown in the graphs. The Excel® sheets listing the data from the eight papers are available at the website **Open Science Framework** (https://osf.io) in the public project entitled "Appendix for Hidden Data". The Bates stamped documents containing data and, in many cases, protocols, are also accessible there.

In most cases, experiments took 11 or 12 days to complete from start to finish. I made sure that all of the experiments I attribute to each of the papers were completed before the papers were received by the journals either initially, or by the time of acceptance. I note those dates when discussing each paper.

Analyses in this book demonstrate that many of the experiments reported in the eight papers are statistically unsound. I believe this should be acknowledged, and the papers should be retracted as appropriate. I have approached Editors of three of the four journals in which questionable data were published with requests to retract. As of the publication date of this book, none has been willing to do so. Nevertheless, what follows should serve to warn the scientific community that results presented in these papers raise questions as to their reliability.

The articles fall into three groups. The three papers in the first group deal with the effects of radical scavengers on the survival of V79 Chinese hamster cells that have taken up various radionuclides differing in their radiologic properties. The journal *Radiation Research* published two of the papers, and *Acta Oncologica* published the third. The second group of two papers deals with the effects of external beam gamma rays, ^{32}P-orthophosphate and ^{117m}Sn(4+)diethylenetriaminepentaacetic acid on the survival of colony-forming cells derived from treated mice's bone marrow. The *Journal of Nuclear Medicine* published both. The 3rd group contains three papers. Two were published in *Radiation Research* and deal with the bystander effect in V79 cells treated with ^{3}H-thymidine that were co-incubated with non-radioactive cells. I am a co-author on the second of these. The third article was published in the journal *Micron* and deals in a similar fashion with the bystander effect in V79 cells exposed to ^{125}IdU and subsequently co-incubated with untreated (bystander) cells.

Group One: Survival of V79 Chinese Hamster Lung Cells Exposed to Radionuclides in the Presence of the Radical Scavengers Dimethyl Sulfoxide (DMSO) and Cysteamine (MEA)

The radionuclides used in these three papers were ^{3}H$_2$O, ^{125}IdU, ^{131}IdU, all three papers; ^{32}P-orthophophate and ^{3}H-thymidine, Paper One; and ^{210}Polonium citrate, Papers Two and Three. These compounds were chosen for very specific reasons. ^{3}H (tritium, a radioactive isotope of hydrogen), ^{131}I (a radioactive form of iodine) and ^{32}P (a radioactive form of phosphorus) all produce beta particles or rays when they decay. In radioactive decay, the atomic nucleus disintegrates producing distinct sub-atomic particles. Beta particles or beta rays are synonymous with electrons, but they come from atomic nuclei, whereas electrons come from outer atomic shells. The beta rays produced when these three isotopes decay have different energies with ^{32}P being the strongest and ^{3}H being the weakest. When such isotopes decay, they generate a track along which ionizations occur. The longest track is that of ^{32}P and the shortest is that of ^{3}H. The ^{3}H track is so short that its interactions would not go beyond the outer membrane of the cell in which its decay has occurred. ^{3}H$_2$O would rapidly equilibrate with water inside of cells, some molecules would participate in reactions involving water, and the rest would be removed when the cells are washed after exposure. Much of the cellular damage results from proximity to the radionuclide during the exposure. ^{3}H-thymidine, on the other hand, is a precursor of DNA. If the cell is in the process of replicating at the time of exposure, the ^{3}H-thymidine will incorporate into the DNA and when it decays, will damage the molecules in its environment – primarily

DNA. Its decay could be lethal or could produce mutations. The same could be said for ^{131}IdU and ^{125}IdU, which are also radioactive DNA precursors.

When ^{125}I decays, about 7% of the product are gamma rays. (10% of the product from ^{131}I decay are also gamma rays.) The remaining decay products from ^{125}I are 21 Auger electrons of 50 to 500 electron volts (eV) (compare to ^{3}H beta decay energy of 18.6 kilo-electron volts (keV)). This energy would dissipate very locally and could be very damaging.

There are two ways that radiations can interact with matter and -- ultimately – kill cells: by direct effect and by indirect effect. In direct effect interactions, the primary electron resulting from the radiation interacts directly with the target molecules, i.e., with, for example, DNA, causing strand breaks and base damage. So-called high linear energy transfer (LET) radiations (e.g. alpha particles and Auger electrons) act by direct effect. Low LET radiations such as X-, beta and gamma rays act by indirect effect. The first chemical event is the ionization of water that produces a number of active chemical species, the most deleterious of which is the hydroxyl radical, which in its turn damages macromolecules such as DNA. Radical scavengers can mollify indirect effect interactions. Among the best known are DMSO and 2-mercaptoethanolamine (MEA) otherwise known as cysteamine. These radical scavengers are themselves quite toxic to cells, so their concentrations are critical.

These studies are of interest academically because one would predict that the radical scavengers DMSO and MEA would protect against the killing effects of the indirect effect beta-emitters, ^{3}H, ^{131}I and ^{32}P. However, what would be their impact against the high LET radionuclides ^{210}Po and ^{125}I? If these only act directly, the scavengers would have no effect on their activity, but if there is an indirect component, then some protection should be observed.

The first paper in this series, published in *Radiation Research*, studied the effect of 5% DMSO on killing of V79 Chinese hamster cells by ^{32}P-orthophosphate, ^{3}H$_2$O, ^{3}H-thymidine, ^{125}IdU and ^{131}IdU. These radionuclides except for ^{125}IdU contain low LET radioisotopes so DMSO would act as a protector for them. Most of the experiments reported in this paper were performed before

Bishayee joined the Lab. The results showed protection for ^{32}P and $^{3}H_2O$ but not for ^{3}H-thymidine, ^{125}IdU or ^{131}IdU, although protection would be expected for ^{3}H-thymidine and ^{131}IdU, as well. Bishayee only performed the three experiments involving ^{131}IdU. At that time, he had been in the Lab for about 2.5 months and was probably being closely supervised. His results were not inconsistent with the others, and the lack of protection that was observed could be due to the use of 5% DMSO instead of the 10% reported later. When Bishayee's results are broken down by experiment, there is already a suggestion in his second experiment of an unusually high number of averages in the colony triples. In that same experiment, the Coulter terminal digits are not likely to be random, as well (See Table 4).

The second paper, published in *Radiation Research*, again involved DMSO, but here the concentration was 10%, which would be expected to produce better protection than the 5% used in the first studies. The radionuclides were $^{3}H_2O$, ^{125}IdU, ^{131}IdU and ^{210}Po. Bishayee performed all the experiments. Protection was as expected: DMSO reduced killing by $^{3}H_2O$, and both iodine radionuclides but, as predicted, had no effect on ^{210}Po, which interacts by direct effect. Interestingly, there appears to be no reason based on statistical analysis to be suspicious of these ^{210}Po results. On the other hand, the results of test 1 for colonies for the other three radionuclides show a significant lack of randomness.

The third paper, published in *Acta Oncologica*, involves $^{3}H_2O$, ^{125}IdU, ^{131}IdU and ^{210}Po and the protector MEA. There should be protection for $^{3}H_2O$ and ^{131}IdU but not necessarily for ^{125}IdU and ^{210}Po, both of which are high LET. Bishayee performed all of these experiments. MEA was reported to be protective for all four radionuclides, but less so for ^{210}Po. Statistical analysis (Test 1) leads one to question the results for all four radionuclides.

Howell discusses the discrepancy between the ^{210}Po results in the *Acta Oncologica* paper (MEA protection of ^{210}Po) compared to the second *Radiation Research* paper (no DMSO protection of ^{210}Po). He has no explanation for the difference. The ^{210}Po results in the *Acta Oncologica* paper are questionable based on my statistical analysis so the protection by MEA can likely be disregarded. I found three experiments involving DMSO protection of ^{210}Po in the

Discovery materials, but only two are shown in the second *Radiation Research* paper. Analysis of all three results in 9 averages in 30 triples, with 4.64 + 1.96 expected, a Z-value of 1.96 and probability P$\geq$ 9 of 0.032. Table 5 shows six averages in 20 triples, 3.11 expected, probability p$\geq$6 of 0.076. Taken together, it is not at all clear how radical scavengers affect ^{210}Po if one has to rely on these two papers. Bishayee was the investigator in a total of 14 experiments with ^{210}Po found in the Discovery materials. Figure 4F includes results of all of them. The probability for the Mid-Ratio distribution shown therein to be random was less than 10^{-40}.

Statistical Analysis of Experiments in the Group One Papers

Paper #1) Howell RW, Goddu SM, Bishayee A, Rao DV. Radioprotection against lethal damage caused by chronic irradiation with radionuclides *in vitro*. *Radiation Research* 150:391-9 (1998).

The paper was received January 6, 1997 (before Bishayee arrived in the Lab) and was accepted May 21, 1998. Bishayee's experiments (Figure 5) must have been added in the revision. A grant from the National Cancer Institute supported the project in part. Howell cites this paper in the grant #1 and #2 applications and lists it on his *Curricula vitae* that appear in grants #1, #2, #3 applications and the Renewal. This paper has been cited 17 times, most recently in July 2014. Howell himself cited it nine times most recently in August 2004.

There are eight figures in this paper. I found data in the Discovery materials that matched only five of the eight. There are two plots in each of the graphs in Figures 3 through 7 showing survivals of V79 exposed to varying concentrations of different nuclides in the absence and presence of 5% DMSO. The experiments in the four graphs (^{32}P) in Figure 3 performed by Howell were completed by October 1995. The 3 graphs (^{3}H$_2$O) in Figure 4 performed by Howell were completed by February 1997. The 3 graphs (^{131}IdU) in Figure 5 are all in experiments attributed to Bishayee and were begun on 11/13, 12/04 and 12/08/97, respectively. The three experiments each in Figures 6 (^{3}HdThd) and 7 (^{125}IdU) are attributed to a postdoctoral fellow, Li, and to Howell respectively and were completed in July 1996.

No averages appear in the colony triple data of Bishayee's first experiment for Figure 5 while eight averages are present in the second and third experiments, each shown separately in Table 3. There were no Coulter counts recorded for his third experiment, so the numbers recorded in the Coulter Table represent the 1st and 2nd experiments alone. It would seem that Bishayee's numbers were beginning to be erratic about a month after he started working in the Radiation Research Lab.

Colony Counts									Coulter Counts	
Figure	Qual Triples /Total	K=# w Mean	N=# Exp'd	SD	Z-Value	P≥K	Term Dig Chi Sq P	# Term Digits	Term Dig Chi Sq P
3	43/44	8	7.4	2.5	0.1	0.5	0.6	33	0.3
4	29/29	6	4.3	1.9	0.6	0.3	0.7	60	1.0
5(1)	*9/9*	*0*	*1.4*	*1.1*	*-1.7*	*1.0*	*0.6*	*30*	*0.4*
5(2)	*9/10*	*5*	*1.7*	*1.2*	*2.4*	*2.0x10⁻²*	*0.4*	*30*	*2.3x10⁻²*
5(3)	*9/10*	*3*	*1.8*	*1.2*	*0.6*	*0.3*	*2.8x10⁻²*		
5(all)	27/29	8	4.8	2.0	1.3	0.1	4.4x10⁻³	60	3.8x10⁻³
6	29/29	5	5.3	2.1	-0.4	0.6	0.1		0.7
7	30/31	7	6.3	2.2	0.1	0.5	0.8		0.5

Table 4. Analysis of experiments depicted in Figures 3-7 of the first paper. Column 2 shows the triples for which the high minus the low is ≥ 2 (qualifying triples) over the total number of triples. Abbreviations: Qual (qualifying), no. (number); w (with); sd (standard deviation); Prob (probability); Term (terminal). Not shown are Coulter equal terminal pair probabilities that were all greater than 0.4. Bishayee only performed experiments in Figure 5. Data for the 3 graphs in Figure 5 are shown separately in italics. There were no Coulter counts for graph #3.

Paper #2) Bishayee A, Rao DV, Bouchet LG, Bolch WE, Howell RW. Protection by DMSO against cell death caused by intracellularly localized iodine-125, iodine-131 and polonium-210. *Radiation Research* 153: 416-427 (2000).

This paper was received March 8, 1999, and accepted December 23, 1999. All of the experiments were performed between January and November 1998. It has been cited 39 times, most recently in January 2015. Howell has cited the paper eight times, most recently in September, 2007. He lists it on his *Curriculum vitae* in the grant Renewal application and he cites it in the application for grant #2 in the references and in his Biographical Sketch. There is no acknowledgement of support. The paper has five figures. Bishayee performed all of the experiments that I analyzed.

Figure	Isotope	# Exps	Colony Counts							Term Digit Chi sq P	Coulter Counts	
			Qual triples/ Total	K=# w Mean	N =# Exp'd	sd	Z-value	P≥K			# Term Digits	Term Digit Chi sq P
1	^{3}H2O ^{125}IdU ^{131}IdU	6	58/60	20	8.2	2.6	4.3	4.0x10^{-5}	1.0x10^{-3}	177	0.73
2	^{3}H$_2$O	2	20/20	11	2.5	1.5	5.4	6.3x10^{-6}	0.09	60	0.15
3	^{131}IdU	2	20/20	7	3.0	1.6	2.3	2.0x10^{-2}	0.6	60	1.6x10^{-2}
4	^{125}IdU	2	20/20	7	2.9	1.6	2.3	1.8x10^{-2}	1.3x10^{-2}	60	0.3
5	^{210}Po-citrate	2	20/20	6	3.1	1.6	1.5	0.076	0.41	60	0.09
ALL		14	138/140	53	21.2	4.2	7.4	4.6x10^{-11}	1.1x10^{-8}	417	0.2

Table 5. Analysis of the data relating to the graphs in the 5 Figures in the paper. Column headings as listed for Tables 3 and 4.

The Coulter count terminal digits in Figure 3 in the paper are significantly non-uniform. The colony count terminal digits relating to Figures 1 and 4 in the paper are likewise significantly non-uniform. With the exception of ^{210}Po, the occurrence of the means in the triples is more than double the expected (but see above page 33, ^{210}Po P≥K would be 0.032, significant -- not 0.076 -- if the third experiment of this kind were included). In the aggregate, the colony p≥K for Test 1 (4.64x10^{-11}) and the terminal digit Chi squared probability (1.09 x 10^{-8}) suggest that these results are not reliable.

Paper #3) Bishayee A, Rao DV, Howell RW. Radiation protection by cysteamine against the lethal effects of intracellularly localized Auger electron, α- and β-particle-emitting radionuclides. *Acta Oncologica* 39: 713-720 (2000).

The journal acknowledged receipt of this paper on October 18, 1999, and accepted it July 6, 2000. Support was not acknowledged. It has been cited seven times, most recently in

December 2012. Howell cited it twice, most recently in February 2005. There are 5 Figures in the paper. The experiments were performed between March and December 1998; Bishayee was the investigator for all of them.

Figure	Isotope	Colony Counts Qual Triples/ Total	K=# w mean	N=# Exp'd	sd	Z-value	P ≥K	Term Digit Chi sq Prob	Coulter Counts No. Term. Digits	Term Digit Chi sq Prob
1	^3H_2O	20/20	16	2.7	1.5	8.4	$2.5x10^{-11}$	$1.6x10^{-2}$	60	0.3
	^{131}IdU	10/10	5	1.5	1.1	2.7	$8.9x10^{-4}$	0.1	30	$4.4x10^{-4}$
	^{125}IdU	20/20	11	2.9	1.6	4.8	$2.6x10^{-5}$	$7.9x10^{-3}$	60	$9.3x10^{-4}$
	^{210}Po	20/20	15	2.7	1.5	7.7	$7.0x10^{-10}$	0.3	60	0.1
1	ALL	70/70	47	9.9	2.9	12.7	$2.6x10^{-24}$	$3.0x10^{-6}$	210	$1.4x10^{-3}$
2	^3H_2O	20/20	11	3.0	1.6	4.7	$3.4x10^{-5}$	0.1	60	0.3
3	^{131}IdU	30/30	11	5.1	2.1	2.6	$7.5x10^{-3}$	$4.3x10^{-3}$	90	0.3
4	^{125}IdU	20/20	7	3.6	1.7	1.7	0.54	0.6	60	0.9
5	^{210}Po	30/30	13	4.9	2.0	3.8	$3.9x10^{-4}$	0.1	90	0.3
Fig 1-5	TOTAL	170/170	89	26.5	4.7	13.2	$4.1x10^{-29}$	$3.7x10^{-9}$	510	0.1

Table 6. Analysis of experiments depicted in the Figures in *Acta Oncologica*. The paper called for two experiments for ^{131}IdU in Figure 1. However, only one was found in the Discovery materials.

Table 6 shows the results of my analysis of the data supporting the figures in this paper. The results in Figure 1 for all four isotopes are undependable, and the same appears true for Figures 2, 3 and 5. The Table does not show the data for mean-containing Coulters in Figure 1. Nevertheless, for ^3H_2O Coulters, there were four mean-containing triples where only 1.03 + 0.99 were expected (Z-value of 2.51, p≥K of $1.73x10^{-2}$). For ^{131}IdU Coulters, there were four mean-containing triples where only 0.61+ 0.76 were expected (Z-value of 3.81, p≥K of $2.19x10^{-3}$). I believe that none of the results reported in this paper can be trusted.

Group Two: Mouse Bone Marrow Colony-forming Units After Injections of Radionuclides and Exposure to External Beam Gamma Rays: A Model for the Alleviation of Bone Pain

Bone-seeking radionuclides can be used to alleviate pain resulting from cancer metastases in the bone. One of the side effects would, of course, be excessive killing of bone marrow cells. Cells from mouse bone marrow are frequently used to study toxic effects of drugs and radiation. The marrow cells can be easily extracted from femurs, counted and plated in soft agar where individual surviving cells will grow into colonies. While the technique is somewhat different from that used to quantify colonies from tissue culture cells, the result is the same and the same statistical distributions of cells in triples is expected.

Statistical Analysis of Experiments in the Group Two Papers

There were nine mouse experiments found in the Discovery materials. Bishayee was the investigator for all. They fall into two distinct groups: the first group of four experiments started on 7/29/98 and ended on 9/7/98 and the second group of five began on 9/14/98 and ended on 10/14/98. The Coulter counts and the colony terminal digits are not irregular and are not shown. Experiments _**1**_ and _**2**_ involved external beam acute ^{137}Cs-irradiation as a surrogate for radionuclide irradiation to the bone. Experiments _**3**_ and _**4**_ involved ^{117m}Sn, an isotope of tin (Sn) that decays by producing fairly low energy "conversion electrons", a form of low LET beta radiation. There were 21 triples in all in experiments _**1**_ through _**4**_; K = 13 of them contained their own means, where N = 4.1 were expected, $p \geq K = 1.2 \times 10^{-5}$. In the ensuing discussion and Table, I hi-light experiments _**1**_ through _**4**_ in bold, underline and italics to signify that I am not confident in those results. The second group of 5 experiments consisted of experiments 5, 6 and 7 with ^{117m}Sn and experiments 8 and 9 with external beam ^{137}Cs chronic irradiation. Of the 29 triples in this group, only 3 contained their means, 5.2 ± 2.0 were expected, $p \geq K = 0.91$. Overall, putting all nine experiments together, there were 16 of 50 triples that contained their means, 9.3 ± 2.7 expected, $p \geq K = 0.014$.

Bishayee's experiments recorded in the figures in the two papers took results from both groups, and some data were reused. His

---

participation in the first paper only involved experiments _1_ and _2_, the first two ^{137}Cs experiments, and are presented in Figure 8 as inverted triangles. Statistical analysis of these data is shown in Table 7. The $p \geq K = 0.012$ is significant.

Table 7 also shows the experiments called on in the various figures in the second paper. Figures 3 and 4 of the second paper depict [117m]Sn experiments, with the squares in figure 3 taken from experiment _3_ and the circles taken from experiment 5. Figure 4 calls on data taken from experiments _3_, _4_, 6 and 7. Figure 5, ^{137}Cs-external beam chronic irradiation, represents data from experiments 8 and 9. Thus, Figures 3 and 4 rely on some questionable data while Figure 5 results may be genuine.

I conclude that the results attributed to Bishayee in these two papers and included in four of the figures should be considered problematic and potentially unreliable.

Paper #4.) Goddu SM, Bishayee A, Bouchet LG. Bolch WE, Rao DV, Howell RW. Marrow toxicity of [33]P- versus ^{32}P-orthophosphate: Implications for Therapy of Bone Pain and Bone Metastases. N*uclear Medicine* 41:941-951 (2000).

The journal received this paper on March 3, 1999, and accepted it after revision on September 14, 1999. Roger W Howell, Ph.D. is listed as the corresponding author. It is cited in the grant Renewal and grant #3 applications and is listed in Howell's corresponding Biographical Sketches. Some of the support for the research also came from grants from the National Cancer Institute and the Department of Energy. As of August 2015, it has been cited 19 times, most recently earlier in 2015. Four citations were self-citations by Howell. He cited it most recently in February 2010.

Of the eight figures in this paper, Figures 1-5 deal with ^{32}P and [33]P. I did not find any animal experiments with those nuclides in the Discovery material. Figure 6 involves chronic irradiation of the mice using the ^{137}Cs external beam but the survivals in the figure did not match survivals in the nine experiments in the Discovery material. Figure 7 is a diagram. Bishayee appears only to have contributed to Figure 8 (see Table 7 below).

The Coulter counts associated with the experiments in both papers 4 and 5 were blood counts. The terminal digit distributions (not shown) were not significantly different from uniform and there is no reason for concern.

Paper #5. Bishayee A, Rao DV, Srivastava SC, Bouchet LG, Bolch WE, Howell RW. Marrow-sparing effects of $^{117m}Sn(4+)$diethylenetriaminepentaacetic acid for radionuclide therapy of bone cancer. *Nuclear Medicine* 41:2043-2050 (2000)

The journal received this paper on December 28, 1999, and accepted it May 30, 2000. Roger W Howell, Ph.D. is listed as the corresponding author. The National Cancer Institute and the Department of Energy both provided some of the research support. Some of the work was performed at the Brookhaven National Laboratory under contract with the US Department of Energy. It has been cited 39 times, but not by Howell, although he does cite it in the grant Renewal application and in the grant #3 application where he also lists it in his Biographical Sketch.

There are five figures in the paper. Figure 1 has to do with the clearance of tin radioactivity from three mouse tissues; figure 2 has to do with the uptake of radioactivity in the femur. There were no experiments in the Discovery material that corresponded to these two figures. Figure 3 contains two graphs consistent with Bishayee's experiments 4 and 5. Figure 4 has five different symbols on the single plot. I was able to identify data from Bishayee's experiments 3 (open and closed circles), 4, closed triangle, 6, closed diamonds and 7, open squares. Table 7 below shows the Results of my analyses. Figures 3 (squares) and Figure 4 raise serious questions regarding the reliability of the results that are each in part significantly different from random.

	Figure	Symbol	Agent	Exper Nos.	Qual Triples /Total	K=# w Mean	N=# expected	sd	Z-value	P≥K
1st Paper	8	inverted triangle	^{137}Cs	*1,2*	12/12	7	3.0	1.5	2.4	1.2x10^{-2}
2nd Paper	3	Square	^{117m}Sn	*4*	4/4	3	0.5	0.6	3.2	5.5x10^{-3}
	3	Circle	^{117m}Sn	5	5/5	0	1.2	1.0	-1.7	1.00
	4	5 different	^{117m}Sn	*3,4*,6,7	19/19	7	3.0	1.6	2.2	2.0x10^{-2}
	5	circle	^{137}Cs	8,9	12/12	1	2.1	1.3	-1.2	0.90
Both Papers	ALL				52/52	18	9.5	2.7	2.9	3.3x10^{-3}

Table 7. Analysis of colonies from 9 experiments by Bishayee depicted in 4 figures in the two articles. In the calculations for "Both Papers", data that are reused in Figures 3 and 4 are also repeated in the calculations. Questionable experiments *1-4* shown in **bold**, *italics* and underline.

Group Three: Bystander Effects Resulting from Tritiated Thymidine and ^{125}IdU Exposure of Hamster Cells

Bystander effects in cell biology are outcomes, such as death and mutation that occur in cells that were not directly exposed to the toxic agent in question but were within range of cells so exposed. As related to ionizing radiation, bystander effects fall into 2 categories: 1.) those in which the damaged (hit) cell physically contacts neighboring cells that were not directly hit; and 2.) those in which the damaging signal is transmitted to the target cells a distance away through the medium[6]. Such effects have been known for a long time, but interest was heightened for radiation in 1992 when Nagasawa and Little demonstrated that a beam of high LET alpha particles that traversed 1% of tissue culture cells in a dish produced chromosomal damage of a form known as sister chromatid exchanges in about 30% of the cells in the dish.[7] Since that time, the bystander effect has been the focus of intense investigation for radiation biologists for the past 20 years or so.

Chemicals that inhibit cell-cell contact also inhibit bystander effects of the first kind. One such drug is the garden insecticide, lindane. Cells establish contact via the formation of channels between themselves termed gap-junctions. Lindane disrupts such contacts inhibiting bystander effects that depend on gap junction integrity.

The agents transmitting the bystander effect are thought to be reactive-oxygen-species (ROS) and/or free-radicals created in the hit cells and translocated to the bystanders. ROS and free radicals are extinguished by so-called radical-scavengers the archetype for which is the chemical solvent DMSO. Both lindane and DMSO inhibit bystander effects in irradiated human fibroblasts, [8] suggesting that cell-cell contact and ROS are involved. Two of the papers in Group 3, numbers 6 and 7, imply this, as well. They claim to demonstrate that both DMSO and lindane interfere with bystander killing in Chinese hamster V79 cells and that the effects of the two compounds are additive. This may be a lucky guess as Hu et al. also found that both lindane and DMSO reduced bystander effects in an alpha particle model. [9] Bystander effects in Chinese hamster ovary cells can also be transmitted through the culture medium. [10] This bystander mechanism would not be inhibited by lindane.

Understanding the mechanisms of action of bystander effects is important in both diagnostic radiation and therapy. Exploitation of bystander effects in radiation therapy could be used to reduce radiation damage to healthy cells in the vicinity of tumors or to enlarge the effective radiation field without increasing the dose. Likewise, nuclear medicine, which has a role in both diagnosis and treatment, could be tuned more precisely given greater understanding of the role of radiation on the bystanders.

The two papers involving tritiated thymidine have had a significant impact on the radiation research community as the total citations number 196. Thirty-three of these are self-citations by Howell himself.

The experiments in the Radiation Research Lab that involve the bystander effect fall into three categories. 100% experiments are those in which all (i.e. 100%) of the cells in the experiments have been exposed to tritiated thymidine for 12 hours, the time it takes V79 cells to traverse the cell cycle. They are washed free of the unincorporated radionuclide, compacted -- lightly centrifuged – these are now called "clusters". In 50% experiments, half the cells are 100% cells, and the other half (bystanders) were incubated for 12 hours without any radioisotope. Similarly, 10% experiments involve clusters of 10% radioactively exposed cells and 90% unexposed bystander cells. Clusters are incubated for three days in the cold to allow for radioactive decay in the exposed cells. In some experiments, during the three-day incubation, some of the clusters in the incubation tubes in the cold contain DMSO to scavenge ROS, or lindane, to inhibit gap junctions or both.

Paper #6.) Bishayee A, Rao DV, Howell RW. Evidence for pronounced bystander effects caused by nonuniform distributions of radioactivity using a novel three-dimensional tissue culture model. *Radiation Research* 152:88-97 (1999).

The Journal received the paper on March 31, 1999, and accepted it on May 6, 1999. Bishayee completed the last experiment on March 29, 1999. The paper was cited in the grant application and the Renewal and was featured on the cover of the journal issue in which it appeared. It has been cited 95 times since publication, most recently in March of 2015. Howell has cited it 21 times most recently in January 2013. No support is acknowledged, but all three co-authors had appointments at the NJ Medical School and were, therefore, supported, at least in part, by public funds from the state of NJ.

This paper was the first report to claim a bystander effect for incorporated radioactivity and must have been instrumental in awarding the NCI grant (grant #1) to Howell for five years, starting July 1, 2000. It was cited 14 times in the grant application, nine in the Preliminary Studies section. The Renewal provided an additional four years of funding. This paper was cited seven times in the Renewal application (which would have been submitted to the NIH in the fall of 2005, two years after the filing of the *qui tam* suit).

There are eight figures in this first paper. Figure 1 is a diagram and Figure 8 is a photomicrograph. The remaining figures are graphs, and I was able to identify data in the Discovery materials that matched all of them. Figure 2 has two graphs, open diamonds for chronic and closed diamonds for acute irradiation with external beam ^{137}Cs.   Figure 3 also has two graphs, survivals of cells exposed to tritiated thymidine: open and closed diamonds for two 100%, and open and closed circles for two 50% cluster experiments.   Figure 4 records V79 survivals as a function of dose of lindane in the clusters (no radioactivity).   Figure 5 is a lindane dose-response for the "rescue" of bystander cells in 50% clusters. There are three experiments represented in each of figure 4 and figure 5. In fact, these data came from only three experiments. Each experiment had five samples with lindane alone and five samples with lindane plus tritiated thymidine.   Figure 6 has three graphs of each of 2 experiments, all representing 50% tritiated thymidine survivals in clusters.   One graph is a control of tritiated thymidine survival alone (same data as in Figure 3). A second is another control of tritiated thymidine plus 0.58% DMSO (used as a solvent for lindane), and a third is tritiated thymidine plus 0.58% DMSO plus 100 µM lindane. Figure 7 represents conditions for clusters similar to figure 6 except that the clusters consist of 100% cells exposed to tritiated thymidine, as opposed to 50%.

Table 8 below is an analysis of the data that appeared in the six figures in the paper representing experiments found in the Discovery material.   The probabilities, $P \geq K$, for the colony counts are all less than 0.05 and, except for Figure 2, they are all less than 10^{-8}.   The colony terminal digits are significantly non-random for the data represented in Figures 3 and 6. The ALL probability for random or uniform terminal digits of the colony counts is less than 0.001, a figure that would rank as highly significant.   The Coulter terminal digit counts except for Figure 6 are uniformly distributed.

			Colonies							Coulters	
Fig	no. Exps	Exp	Qual Triples/ Total	K=no. w mean	N=no. exp'ed	sd	Z-value	P≥K	Term Digit Chi sq Prob	No. Term. Digits	Term Digit Chi sq Prob
2	2	^{137}Cs Survival	16/16	7	2.9	1.5	2.3	1.6×10^{-2}	0.59	48	0.47
3	4	50% 100%	39/39	26	6.1	2.3	8.6	6.4×10^{-13}	8.7×10^{-3}	120	0.89
4	3	Lindane	15/15	11	1.8	1.3	7.0	4.6×10^{-11}	0.32	45	0.10
5	3	Lindane Survival	15/15	15	2.4	1.4	8.6	2.8×10^{-16}	0.26	45	0.10
6	6	50%	59/59	43	8.6	2.7	12.5	7.0×10^{-24}	4.7×10^{-3}	180	4.1×10^{-12}
7	5	100%	55/60	32	11.5	3.0	6.7	1.2×10^{-9}	0.21	162	0.05
ALL	23		169/174	108	29.1	4.9	16.1	3.4×10^{-42}	1.6×10^{-4}	600	3.9×10^{-8}

Table 8. Colony and Coulter count analysis of data in experiments reported in the first tritiated thymidine paper.   Bishayee performed all the experiments.

Paper #7) Bishayee A, Hill HZ, Stein D, Rao DV, Howell RW. Free-radical-initiated and gap junction-mediated bystander effect due to nonuniform distribution of incorporated radioactivity in a three-dimensional tissue culture model. *Radiation Research* 155:335-344 (2001).

The journal received the paper on July 17, 2000, and accepted it on October 6, 2000.   Howell is the corresponding author. Two grants from the DHHS provided support, one of which was Grant #1 analyzed above. Bishayee completed the final experiment on March 6, 2000.   It has been cited 101 times since it was published, most recently in March 2015.   Howell has cited it 12 times, most recently in December 2012. This paper was cited in the grant Renewal application and on his Biographical Sketch therein.

Figures 1 depict three plots of 100% survivals of V79 cells under three conditions: clusters with and without DMSO and suspensions without DMSO. Figure 2A depicts 50% experiments and has four plots: 1.) no additives, 2.) DMSO, 3.) lindane, and 4.) DMSO and lindane during the cold incubations.   Figure 2B depicts 10% experiments under the same four conditions. Figure 3 is a time study of radioactivity incorporation per cell. The findings in this paper, if true, would be important. The paper claims to demonstrate that the bystander effect (the death of non-radioactive cells in the presence of radioactive cells) requires cell-cell contact via gap junctions. In fact, Vines et al.[10] showed that bystander effects in Chinese hamster cells do not require cell-cell contact. The lethal factor(s) can travel through the medium bathing the cells.

Table 9 shows the statistical analyses for this report. In the three graphs in Figure 1, 55 of 103 qualifying colony triples contain their means, with only 17.1 expected for a probability of $\leq 2.1 \times 10^{-22}$. The corresponding Coulter count terminal digits were also unlikely to be random ($p = 4.1 \times 10^{-3}$). Figure 2 is of even greater concern. In 2A, there are 91 mean-containing triples, 20.8 expected (probability 4.2×10^{-61}) and in 2B, 60 mean-containing triples, 12.1 expected (probability 2.3×10^{-48} expected). Randomness or uniformity for the Coulter terminal digits is also highly unlikely for Figure 2 ($p = 2.1 \times 10^{-27}$ for 2A, and $p = 3.1 \times 10^{-28}$ for 2B).

In Table 9, I show for Figures 1 and 2, for the first time, the Test 1 analysis of the Coulter counts because the average appeared in these triples at a considerably higher rate than expected. Likewise, in Figure 2B, there is a high rate of occurrence of terminal doubles in the Coulter counts, so the column showing this for all the figures is included as well. This is the first paper for which Coulter terminal doubles are significantly more frequent than expected.

I conclude that the results depicted in Figures 1 and 2 are very unlikely to have occurred by chance. Furthermore, as I will demonstrate below, the exponential survivals illustrated in these Figures are contrary to expectation based on biochemical and radiobiological principles. I expected the survival kinetics to have been biphasic, but here survival is represented in all cases by an exponential decline with no change in slope (see chapter 8, Figure 8).

Colonies

Figure	No. Exps	Exp	Symbol	Qual Triples	N = # w Mean	K=# Expected	sd	Z-Value	P≥K	Term Digit Chi sq Prob
1	8	100%	Open Circle	65/67	36	11.1	3.00	8.14	4.1x10^-15	5.9x10^-3
	4		Closed Circle	24/24	11	3.61	1.74	3.96	1.9x10^-4	0.12
	2		Square	14/14	8	2.41	1.39	3.65	5.9x10^-4	0.95
	14		ALL	103/105	55	17.1	3.74	10.01	2.1x10^-22	4.1x10^-3
2A	3	50%	Triangle	27/27	19	4.17	1.87	7.68	2.4x10^-13	0.12
	3		Square	27/27	20	4.10	1.85	8.31	1.2x10^-15	0.30
	4		Diamond	37/37	25	5.67	2.17	8.67	7.5x10^-17	0.40
	5		Circle	42/43	22	6.90	2.38	8.23	2.5x10^-15	0.092
	14		ALL	133/134	91	20.8	4.16	16.74	4.2x10^-61	1.1x10^-3
2B	2	10%	Triangle	20/20	15	2.94	1.58	7.33	3.6x10^-12	0.16
	2		Square	20/20	14	2.99	1.58	6.64	3.5x10^-10	0.15
	2		Diamond	20/20	18	3.15	1.62	8.88	1.6x10^-17	0.57
	2		Circle	20/20	13	3.01	1.59	5.96	2.0x10^-8	0.08
	8		ALL	80/80	60	12.1	3.18	14.9	2.3x10^-48	6.1x10^-4

Coulters

Fig	No. Exps	Exp	Symbol	Qual Triples	N = # w Mean	K=# Expected	sd	Z-value	P≥K	Term Digit Chi sq Prob	Equal Term Pair
1	8	100%	Open Circle	69/69	7	4.29	2.00	1.10	0.14	0.48	0.60/20
	4		Closed Circle	34/34	8	2.09	1.40	3.86	4.0x10^-4	6.5x10^-4	0.32/12
	2		Square	14/14	1	0.87	0.90	-0.41	0.61	0.17	0.93/2
	14		ALL	117/117	16	7.26	2.61	3.16	2.1x10^-3	2.0x10^-3	0.60/34
2A	3	50%	Triangle	25/25	2	1.37	1.14	0.11	0.40	4.6x10^-3	0.13/11
	3		Square	27/27	5	1.45	1.17	2.60	1.5x10^-2	2.7x10^-5	0.11/12
	4		Diamond	37/37	4	2.44	1.51	0.70	0.23	5.5x10^-16	6.8x10^-3/20
	5		Circle	44/44	9	2.73	1.60	3.61	8.0x10^-4	6.8x10^-6	0.34/15
	14		ALL	133/133	20	7.99	2.74	4.20	6.6x10^-5	2.1x10^-27	2.6x10^-3/58
2B	2	10%	Triangle	20/20	0	1.21	1.07	-1.60	0.97	3.4x10^-7	1.5x10^-2/12
	2		Square	20/20	5	1.20	1.06	3.10	4.8x10^-3	6.9x10^-7	1.5x10^-2/12
	2		Diamond	20/20	2	1.17	1.05	0.31	0.33	2.0x10^-4	3.4x10^-2/11
	2		Circle	20/20	3	1.29	1.10	1.11	0.14	1.7x10^-7	7.3x10^-2/10
	8		ALL	80/80	10	4.87	2.14	2.17	2.5x10^-2	3.1x10^-28	2.9x10^-3/45
3	2	Tritium Activity	Circles	26/26	2	0.84	0.90	0.74	0.21	0.36	0.38/9

Table 9. Statistical analysis of graphs in the three figures in the 2nd tritiated thymidine paper. The upper value in the "Equal Terminal Pair", the last column, is the binomial probability for the pair occurrence, the lower value is the number of pair occurrences in the dataset. To determine the number of counts in the terminal pair calculation, multiply the denominator in the Coulter Qual Triples column by 3.

Paper #8.) Howell RW. Bishayee, A. Bystander effects caused by nonuniform distributions of DNA-incorporated [125]I. *Micron* 33:127-132 (2002)

The third paper in this group involves bystander effects of radioactive iodine.

Micron describes itself as "The International Research and Review Journal for Microscopy", but, curiously, this paper has nothing to do with microscopy. Howell and Bishayee's paper was included in a special issue of the journal devoted to the "Biological effects of radiation: role of electron microscopy". M. Tzaphlidou, a professor of Medicine in the Laboratory of Medical Physics in the Medical School of the University of Ioannina in Greece was the Editor. Dr Tzaphlidou appears to be mainly interested in collagen, not, as far as I know, a particular interest of either Bishayee or Howell. Possibly Howell came to know her at meetings they both attended or somehow through a connection with the now called Society of Nuclear Medicine and Molecular Imaging. Howell notes in his *curriculum vitae* that this paper was INVITED.

[125]I, the radionuclide featured in this study, has interesting properties with respect to decay that involves the production of Auger electrons. These occur in large numbers (about 20 per decay) and dissipate their energy very locally, somewhat like sparklers on the 4th of July, in contrast to fireworks. [125]IdU is an analog of thymidine and incorporates into DNA. The decay of ^{125}I thus results in lethal damage with the same force as an alpha particle. Although it produces electrons that are low energy, their production in a small cloud can be very deleterious. In fact, studies have shown that [125]IdU is considerably more lethal to cells in culture than either [131]IdU or ^{3}H-thymidine[11]. When ^{125}I is delivered to the cytoplasm and not to the nucleus, its effects are far less lethal. It has been the hope that ^{125}I and other Auger-producing nuclides will be effective in cancer therapy. The purpose of this report as defined in the paper's Introduction is to examine the presence and extent of any bystander effect resulting from the incorporation of [125]IdU into the DNA of V79 cells.

The article does not state the submission date of the paper to the journal, but it became available in PubMed Central in February 2001, and on-line in September 2001. It was supported by two

DHHS grants. Howell was the Principal Investigator on one (grant #1 above), and the other was a shared instrument grant with Thomas Denny as Principal Investigator. Howell cited it in the grant Renewal application and also listed it in his Biographical Sketch. As of August 1, 2015, it has been cited 31 times, most recently in September 2014. There are twelve self-citations by Howell, the most recent of which is September 2014.

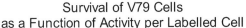

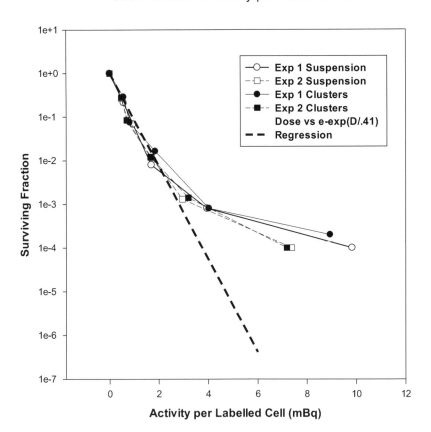

Figure 6. After Figure 1 in the *Micron* paper but representing all the Discovery data in the two experiments. The figure in the *Micron* paper does not show data beyond 4 mBq. The dashed line in this figure is calculated using the value of 0.41mBq/labeled cell listed in Table 1 of the *Micron* paper for 100% cells labeled.

I found two experiments in the Discovery materials that correspond to the two plots in Figure 1 of the paper. I plotted the data myself, as shown in my Figure 6. My results (my Figure 6, symbols) are very similar to those in the paper, at least up to 4 mBq per labelled cell. However, my plots constructed from the two Discovery experiments continue beyond the plots in the paper and indicate a distinct change in slope after 4 mBq per labelled cell.

C. G. Bagley posed six questions that "every author, editor, reviewer and reader should ask themselves when evaluating a research paper". His question #3 is "Were all the results presented? Inappropriate data selection is a crucial issue."[12] I posit that withholding the information regarding the change in slope is potentially a critical issue that could alter the interpretation of results in the second *Micron* figure. At the very least, all three plots in *Micron* Figure 2 should be biphasic, as their kinetics depend on the survival kinetics shown in my Figure 6.

In my Figure 6, I also show the theoretical survival based on the value of A_1 of 0.41mBq/labelled cell (dashed line) recorded in Table 1 of the *Micron* paper. Table 1 in the paper does not reflect the biphasic nature of the slope that must occur, as per my Figure 6, with higher input radioactivity. This, again, withholds information from the reader.

Table 10 below raises additional concerns with respect to statistical analyses of the two data sets in the two experiments depicted in my Figure 6 (and in *Micron* Figure 1). The p-values for uniformity of terminal digits of both Coulter and colony counts recorded for the cells in suspension are significant as is the occurrence of equal terminal pairs. There is no discernable problem with the clusters.

The primary concern for Figure 1 in the paper has to do with information that was withheld. As for Figure 2, it is quite a different story. The data supporting all three graphs appear to have problems regarding both the P$\geq$K for colonies and the terminal digits for Coulter counts.

				Colonies						
Figure	No. Exps.	Exp	Symbols	Qual Triples/Total	K=# w Mean	N=# Expected	sd	Z-Value	P≥K	Term Dig Chi Sq P
1	2	clusters	closed	13/14	4	3.0	1.5	0.3	0.4	0.4
	2	Suspension	open	12/14	5	2.9	1.5	1.1	0.1	0.026
	4		ALL	25/28	9	5.9	2.1	1.3	0.1	0.039
2	6	100%	Circles	48/50	26	10.0	2.8	5.6	6.2×10^{-8}	8.5×10^{-3}
	6	50%	Triangles	51/51	31	9.1	2.7	8.0	3.3×10^{-12}	0.19
	4	10%	Diamonds	34/34	19	5.4	2.1	6.2	7.2×10^{-8}	0.14
	16		ALL	133/135	76	24.5	4.4	11.7	4.0×10^{-30}	2.0×10^{-4}

Figure	No. Exps.	Exp	Symbols	Coulters No. Term. Digits	Term DigitChi sq Prob	Equal Term Pair/#pairs
1	2	clusters	closed	42	0.9	0.054/8
	2	Suspension	open	42	2.6×10^{-2}	0.021/9
	4		ALL	84	0.08	3.6×10^{-3}/17
2	6	100%	Circles	153	8.7×10^{-12}	0.052/22
	6	50%	Triangles	153	7.2×10^{-17}	9.8×10^{-3}/25
	4	10%	Diamonds	102	2.9×10^{-11}	0.04716
	16		ALL	408	1.8×10^{-43}	3.8×10^{-4}/63

Table 10: Analysis of Experimental Data for *Micron* Figures 1 and 2. Figure 2 in the paper calls for data from four 100% experiments. However, I found six such experiments and could not determine which were the four depicted in the paper. I have, therefore, included data from all 6. Just to be sure I was being fair, I recalculated the 100% results eliminating the 2 experiments that had the highest number of means in the triples. In that case, the P≥K value for colonies increased from 6.20×10^{-8} to 2.74×10^{-3} and the terminal digit Chi square probability increased from 8.47×10^{-3} to 6.38×10^{-3}. The Coulter terminal digit Chi square increased from 8.66×10^{-12} to 2.78×10^{-7} and the equal terminal pair probability decreased from 5.28×10^{-2} for 22 terminal pairs to 2.46×10^{-2} for 17 terminal pairs.

The eight papers from the Radiation Research Lab co-authored by Howell and Bishayee published between October 1998 and February 2001 have been cited 353 times. This drops to 285 times by eliminating self-citations by Howell. These citations are a measure of the interest in the radiation biology world evoked by the topics represented. The three bystander papers (#'s 6, 7 and 8) have been cited 184 times by outside investigators. The favorable priority score that was given to the grant #1 application -- it may well have been the highest ranked submission in the Radiation Study Section -- reflects even further the enthusiasm for this work. Howell has continued to cite papers co-authored with Bishayee as recently as February, 2016, an indication that he still relied on them up to that time. Apparently his support of Bishayee did not waiver in spite of the opinions of my two experts and the failure of his expert to cite three key experiments that refute his arguments.

NB. Chapters 8 – 10 will be of interest mainly to Radiation Biologists.

8. THE TRITIATED THYMIDINE PROBLEM

If the facts don't fit the theory, change the facts

Albert Einstein

100% Tritiated Thymidine Experiments and the Role of Deoxycytidine[*]

Concentrations of thymidine approximately 1 millimolar or greater in tissue culture medium block the cell cycle at the G1/S interface and during S phase.[13,14] Radiation blocks the cell cycle mainly in G2.[14] High specific activity tritiated thymidine blocks the cell cycle and kills cells at nanomolar thymidine concentrations.[15,16,17,18] Deoxycytidine reverses the cell cycle blocking-effect of thymidine.[19,20,21,22,23]

The specific activity of a radionuclide is defined as the radiation dose per unit of mass (e.g. Becquerel/gram or Becquerel/mol). When the specific activity is high, the chemical amount of the nuclide to achieve a given amount of radiation dose is correspondingly small. In seeking an effect from radioactivity alone, it would be desirable to utilize the highest specific activity possible to reduce or eliminate effects due to the chemical itself. The highest available specific activity for tritiated thymidine was used in all the experiments in the Radiation Research Lab.

Numerous reports have described the killing effect of tritiated thymidine on cultured mammalian cell survival. Incubation with the isotope continues up to or somewhat beyond the cell cycle time before plating for colonies. Storage under non-growing conditions allows more tritium decay before plating. Survival curves take three forms: (1) monotonic exponential; (2) initial shoulder then exponential; and (3) biphasic – rapid decline in survival, then slower decline or plateau. When exponential killing occurred

---

[*] Much of the material discussed in this chapter appears in our publication in the journal *Publications* (reference #2)

without[11,24,25] or with[25,26,27, 28] a shoulder, presence of deoxycytidine in the medium was stated either directly or indirectly.[25,29, 30] In its absence, the survival curve was biphasic[18,31,32,33,34, 35], although there was one exception.[36]

In six experiments performed in 1992, long before Bishayee's arrival, V79 cells were incubated with increasing doses of high specific activity tritiated thymidine, with and without deoxycytidine for approximately one cell cycle before plating for colonies (Figure 7). Both survival curves are biphasic, but the final plateau with deoxycytidine is approximately 15-fold lower than in its absence, confirming the reversal of the cell cycle blocking of tritiated thymidine by deoxycytidine.

Howell and Lenarczyk performed a total of ten 100% experiments (all cells exposed to tritiated thymidine): 7 experiments involving V79 cells and three experiments with CHO-K1 cells. No deoxycytidine was present. The V79 survival curves were all biphasic, reaching a survival plateau of approximately 0.5, except for one plateau at approximately 0.3 (Figure 8A). Their survival results contrast with Bishayee's exponential decline reported in the two publications numbers 6 and 7, above. The CHO-K1 survival curves are similar but plateau at survival (S/S_o) of approximately 0.3 (data not shown). Howell's and Lenarczyk's V79 results are consistent with V79 biphasic survivals reported by Keprtova and Minarova[34] under similar conditions. Howell's ultimate survival at 5 mBq is approximately 100 times greater than Bishayee's following the same protocol and using the same cell line. This is a major difference.

The defense's expert witness in the *qui tam* case was Ludwig Feinendegen, MD, an expert in nuclear medicine. He argued that radiobiological parameters listed in Tables 1 of both papers 6 and 7 predicted the exponential survival slope that Bishayee reported in published 100% experiments. Further, that high specific activity tritiated thymidine would not perturb or block the cell cycle because the chemical concentration of thymidine would be too low. However, Feinendegen must have discounted the cell cycle-blocking effect of the radioactivity emanating from the tritium. Cell cycle blocking by radiation is a well-known phenomenon. He apparently was unaware of the papers by Keprtova and Minarova[34], Hu, *et al.*[17] and Persaud *et al.*[31]. These all show biphasic survivals on exposure to high specific activity tritiated thymidine in the absence of deoxycytidine. Feinendegen was not shown Dr Pitt's statistical analyses of Bishayee's results that demonstrate the irregular nature of his data. His job as an expert was only to rebut the Robbins report.

Cleaver and Holford found a 10-minute preincubation with 10^{-9} M thymidine (a very low concentration) decreased the incorporation of 2.5×10^{-6} M tritiated thymidine into DNA by 10%.[37] This finding indicates that minute amounts of thymidine do, indeed, perturb the intracellular thymidine pool. The results shown in Figure 7 demonstrate that deoxycytidine does abrogate the blocking of the cell cycle by tritiated thymidine. Feinendegen was aware of these experiments. However, in the documents available to him, they had not been graphed together as I have done. On the graphs that he saw, it would not have been obvious that the survivals were different with and without deoxycytidine.

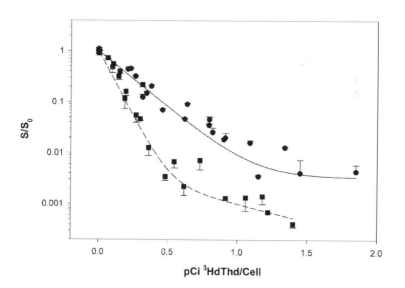

Figure 7. Survival of V79 Cells with and Without Deoxycytidine in the Medium. Survival in the absence of deoxycytidine (circles) and its presence (squares). Experiments performed by post-doctoral fellow R. Harapanhalli. The solid and dashed lines for the survivals were calculated using the Regression Wizard program in the SigmaPlot® graphing software.

The results that are shown in Figure 7 clearly demonstrate that deoxycytidine <u>does</u> affect the survival response of V79 cells exposed to tritiated thymidine, presumably by abrogating, at least to some extent, the thymidine block. Distributions of colony and Coulter counts by all three tests in these six experiments give no cause for concern. However, the survival kinetics displayed in Figure 7 are considerably different from survival kinetics in Howell's and Lenarczyk's 100% experiments. There is good reason for this (see below).

I conclude that experiments available in the literature argue that Howell's and Lenarczyk's 100% experiments (Figure 8A) come close to the expectation and are an accurate representation of tritiated thymidine survivals of V79 cells. Moreover, that Bishayee's survival experiments as presented in the two papers (Nos. 6 and 7) are not compatible with that expectation.

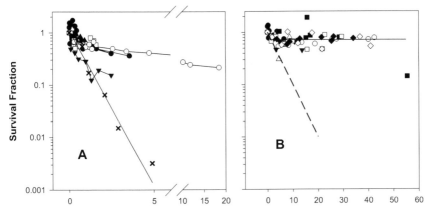

Figure 8. Graphs of unpublished experiments performed by Lenarczyk and Howell following protocols for exposure of 100% (**A**) and 50% (**B**) of V79 cells to tritiated thymidine (©Hill and Pitt[2]). In **A**, the X-X survival curve is the approximate survival calculated using the cross-section A_1 listed in Table 1 of paper 7; the circles represent 2 experiments performed by Howell; the remaining symbols are from 5 experiments performed by Lenarczyk. In **B**, the circles and inverted solid triangles are from 3 experiments performed by Howell, the remaining symbols are from 5 experiments performed by Lenarczyk. The solid line represents a survival of 0.72, the average of survivals for incorporated activities greater than 9 mBq/labelled cell. The dashed line is the approximate survival curve estimated from 50% survivals in papers 6 and 7, above.

Fifty Percent Experiments and the Bystander Effect

In papers 6 and 7, Bishayee and Howell claim to be first to show a bystander effect using incorporated radioactivity, i.e. tritiated thymidine. They also claim that the bystander effect is abrogated by DMSO, a scavenger of reactive oxygen species (ROS) and by lindane, an inhibitor of gap junction intracellular communication (GJIC). Therefore, they conclude that the bystander effect is transmitted by cell-to-cell communication involving the transfer of ROS from one cell to another. However, others have shown that bystander effects in CHO cells are transmitted through the medium[10] and do not require cells to communicate. Bystander effects in radiation impact both radiation therapy and nuclear medicine[38,39]. Inaccurate information could lead to errors in treatment planning, in allowable doses in diagnostic nuclear medicine and permissible workplace exposures.

Figure 8A shows that there are 100 fold more survivors at about 5 mBq/labeled cell in Lenarczyk's and Howell's 100% experiments than in Bishayee's 100% experiments. Similarly, there are 70-times more survivors at about 20 mBq/labeled cell in Lenarczyk's and Howell's 50% experiments than in Bishayee's 50% experiments. These differences are not trivial; they are significant.

In papers 6 and 7, the authors claim that the purported bystander effect is abrogated by DMSO, lindane and more so by the two together. However, the results in Figure 8B suggest that there is little or no bystander effect under these experimental conditions. If this is true, then there can be no effect of DMSO, lindane or the two together.

Investigators at Columbia University using CHO cells closely related to V79 cells showed that their 100% cells incubated with tritiated thymidine tended toward a plateau of about 30%[31]. Their conditions were slightly, but, importantly, different from those in the Lenarczyk and Howell experiments. Their experiments support Howell's and Lenarczyk's results, but not survivals recorded in papers 6 and 7.

9. THE HELENA TUBES ARE HYPOXIC

It's important for scientists to be a bit less arrogant, a bit more humble, recognizing we are capable of making mistakes and being fallacious

Robert Winston

Hypoxic conditions decrease the lethal effects of low linear energy transfer (LET) radiation (tritium (beta), gamma and X-rays) by up to approximately 3-fold; this is the so-called "oxygen effect."[13] The "clusters" that were assembled for most of the experiments that I analyzed from the Radiation Research Lab consisted of pellets of 4 million cells loosely lying at the bottom of narrow plastic tubes (Helena tubes) with a capacity 0.4 ml. The tubes were filled to the brim with culture medium and capped, leaving little or no airspace above the medium. These clusters were incubated at 10.5° centigrade for 72 hours. Under these conditions, the cells would not replicate, but they could still metabolize, albeit more slowly than at 37° Centigrade (the standard incubator temperature, which is equal to the human body temperature). These conditions would be likely to lead to oxygen depletion and, ultimately, hypoxia. The simplest way of determining whether this was conducive to hypoxia would be to measure the oxygen concentration in the tubes with time using an oxygen electrode, a simple, relatively inexpensive device. This was, to my knowledge, never done.

Howell designed the following experiment that did not involve incorporated radioactivity to test the clusters for hypoxia. Aliquots of cells in Helena tubes were incubated in the cold. After 72 hours of cold incubation, cells in five tubes were left undisturbed, hence potentially hypoxic. The cells in the other five tubes were re-aerated by re-suspending and mixing with a pipette, a method used frequently to mix and suspend cells in tubes of medium. This discussion pertains only to the induction of mutations in the undisturbed tubes of clusters that were then exposed to incremental doses of gamma rays. Additional ramifications of this experiment will be described below. I measured mutations in the clusters as a function of dose in the first run of this experiment, and Bishayee repeated my experiment in the second run. Others have shown that hypoxic conditions significantly reduce mutation induction.[40]

In my hands, no mutations were induced in the undisturbed, putative hypoxic, clusters. On the contrary, when Bishayee performed the experiment, he reported significant mutation induction with increasing dose in the intact clusters. Figure 9 left graph compares our two results. It would have been prudent to resolve this conflict by repeating the experiment under close observation by an outside observer, but, to my knowledge, this has not been done. Bishayee's version of the experiment (circles) was presented in Figure 7 of Howell's successful grant application, see above Table 3 on pages 27 to 28.

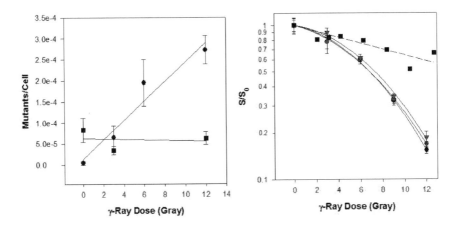

Figure 9. Left: Mutant induction by gamma rays in V79 cells irradiated in clusters. Circles, Bishayee's experiment: 59-fold increase over background at 1200 cGray; Squares, my experiment: 25% decrease from the background at 1200 cGray. There is no discernable difference in protocols between the two experiments. **Right:** V79 survivals in 60 mm tissue culture dishes (circles, three experiments performed by me) and in clusters (squares, 1 experiment performed by Lenarczyk (unpublished). The 60 mm dishes are generally assumed to be well aerated.

In Bishayee's experiment, mutation testing employed 120 Coulter data counts; the terminal digit analysis for uniformity determined a chi-squared p-value of 1.5×10^{-11} for his counts. By way of comparison, I had 65 Coulter data counts for the same purpose with terminal digit p-value of 0.05. There were no additional repetitions of this experiment found in the Discovery documents.

Figure 9, right, compares three survival experiments with V79 in 60 mm dishes performed by me (circles) with one survival experiment with V79 in the Helena tube clusters performed by Lenarczyk (squares). My cells were well-aerated. The relative resistance of Lenarczyk's cells in clusters suggests that they, on the other hand, were hypoxic, presumably due to the lack of sufficient air in the Helena tubes.

I speculate that the set up – Helena tubes with almost no surface for gas exchange -- for most of the experiments involving clusters was conducive to hypoxia. Howell devised this set up as a proxy for conditions in human tissues which, on average, are not severely hypoxic. I think he missed the mark.

10. POTENTIALLY LETHAL DAMAGE

Moments when lost, can't be found again. They're just gone.

Jenny Han

In Radiation Biology, there is a class of radiation damage known as "Potentially Lethal Damage" that is only expressed under certain circumstances[41]. Cells are allowed to grow to confluence: the dish surface remains covered with cells with edges in contact with each other, a growth-arresting condition known as contact inhibition. The cells are then irradiated, harvested and plated for colonies immediately (immediate plating) or allowed to remain confluent for 6 or 12 hours and then plated for colonies (delayed plating). There will be more colonies (survivors) among the cultures for which plating was delayed.

Harapanhalli's survival curves (Figure 7) in the absence of deoxycytidine (circles) indicate that around 10% or less of the cells are relatively resistant to killing by radiation – cf survival at higher doses. Howell's and Lenarczyk's 100% survival curves show that around 30% of the cells are relatively resistant (Figure 8A). Harapanhalli plated the cells after the 12-hour incubation with tritiated thymidine – immediate plating. Howell and Lenarczyk held their cells in close contact in clusters in the cold for three days before plating – delayed plating. A related experiment found in the Discovery materials performed by Howell and a post-doctoral fellow, W. Li, supports Harapanhalli's immediate plating results. It seems likely that most of the survivors in the Howell-Lenarczyk clusters are the survivors of Potentially Lethal Damage. This could be an ideal system for studying this little-understood phenomenon.

11. HIDDEN DATA MEANS HIDDEN COST

Lost time is never found again...Remember that time is money

Benjamin Franklin

Tissue culture experiments are relatively expensive. Necessary equipment is costly, as are consumable supplies. The Radiation Research Lab was equipped with several incubators for maintaining cultures that required continuous gassing with 95% air/5% carbon dioxide and precise temperature control at 37° C (98.6° F), a temperature-controlled incubator for maintaining cultures at 10.5° C for 3 days, an inverted microscope for examining the growth of cultures and colonies, centrifuges of different capacities and speeds, 2 laminar air flow hoods where work is performed under sterile conditions, 2 fume hoods for safe chemical and radiation containment, a high performance liquid chromatograph for concentrating and purifying radio-chemicals, a Coulter particle counter for counting cells in suspension, a liquid scintillation counter for counting low energy radiation samples, an ordinary refrigerator, a -20° freezer, liquid nitrogen freezers requiring topping up every 3 to 4 weeks with a regularly renewable supply of liquid nitrogen for long-term storage and preservation of cells, rollers for keeping cells in suspension during incubation with radio-isotopes. There were other pieces of equipment available in other labs and core facilities but this list names equipment that was present during Bishayee's time in the Lab. I estimate that equipment and amenities like this would cost upwards of $75,000 to $100,000.

Even though my analyses suggest that many experiments were only carried out on paper, there had to be a semblance of work being done and consumables being consumed or suspicions might be aroused. Culture media had to be made up on a routine basis. This required that bottles be washed and sterilized by autoclave, powdered media purchased from vendors had to be dissolved in ultra-pure water and filter sterilized through disposable sterile plastic filters into the sterile glass bottles. Fetal bovine serum, the most costly constituent of tissue culture media, had to be added under sterile conditions, along with antibiotics. The media bottles had to be stored in the refrigerator and consumed on a regular basis lest it be discovered that they were not turning over.

Cells stored in the liquid nitrogen freezer had to be thawed, seeded in disposable plastic culture flasks and grown to sufficient density for experiments. Each experiment would require a dozen or so plastic disposable Falcon® culture tubes for the initial incubations with radio-chemicals, "Helena" microfuge tubes for transfer to and incubation of cells in the 10.5° incubator, additional Falcon® tubes in which to transfer the cells for washing by centrifugation and then sampling. Sampling would involve three disposable plastic vials for Coulter counting for each experimental point, three disposable plastic vials for radiation counting for each experimental point, a series of three plastic disposable polystyrene or polypropylene tubes to make serial dilutions for each experimental point, three or six plastic 60 mm tissue culture dishes for each experimental point. For an experiment with ten experimental points 2 or 3 tissue culture flasks, 120 to 150 tubes will have been consumed and 30 to 60 plastic disposable tissue culture dishes. Syringes and pipettes would be necessary for breaking up clumps of cells and for liquid transfers. These come in several sizes and are discarded after each use – at least ten syringes and perhaps 100 pipettes would be consumed in a 10 point experiment. Once an experiment has been incubated, and colonies are ready for counting, the plastic culture dishes are removed from the incubator, the medium is poured off, the dishes are washed with phosphate-buffered saline, fixed with alcohol and stained with crystal violet or some other blue stain to enhance visualization of the colonies. The plates are dried. Colonies are counted by marking each on the underside with a Sharpie® as they are counted.

Once an experiment was completed, items containing sufficient radioactivity had to be carefully discarded. Such items were collected in marked containers to be carried off by Radiation Safety workers. The particular nuclide and its activity in the containers had to be estimated and written on the outside. The door to the corridor of the Lab was kept locked at all times and keys were only issued to specifically authorized individuals.

A rough estimate of supplies consumed over the four-year period that Bishayee was in the Lab is $60,000. Bishayee's compensation probably came to around $125,000 to $150,000 for the period. Other salaries to factor in would be those of Lenarczyk, Howell himself, student assistants and university personnel employed in cleaning, radiation monitoring and other activities needed to keep the Lab functioning. Not to mention my salary and my time devoted to this endeavor, or the cost to the university to defend the lawsuit. The University's cost more than matched my out-of-pocket cost of approximately $200,000 for the *qui tam*. They hired the second largest law firm in the state and, where I paid only one lawyer, they paid at least two. All of this is in addition to the grant and Renewal based on data generated by Bishayee. I estimate the lost time, effort and expense to be in the range of $3- to $4-million.

12. HOW IT ALL STARTED

Faith: not wanting to know what truth is
Friedrich Nietzsche

Lenarczyk and I observed what we believed to have been suspicious activity on the part of Bishayee beginning in March 2001. I kept a diary of our observations during this time and the experimental protocol, and concomitant records are in the scanned PDF files obtained in Discovery. Bishayee started an experiment on Monday, March 26, with V79 cells. Lenarczyk believed that Bishayee had used cells from a flask containing mold to initiate that research and conveyed that information to me on Wednesday, March 28. (The presence of mold would have rendered the experiment useless.) My diary and the PDF file for this experiment are the only records in the Discovery documents for this period, although Howell and Bishayee claimed there was another one but were unable to produce it. According to Bishayee's protocol, seven cell samples in Helena tubes should have been placed in the 10.5-degree incubator on Tuesday, March 27, to be incubated until Friday, March 30. Each sample should contain cells of two types: cells that had incorporated tritiated thymidine and were also vitally stained with a fluorescent dye, and cells that contained neither tritiated thymidine nor dye (bystanders).

On Thursday evening, March 29, Bishayee asked for and received a fresh flask of uncontaminated V79 cells from Lenarczyk. The next morning, Lenarczyk and I observed a holder containing seven Helena tubes in the 10.5-degree incubator – consistent with the protocol in the notebook for that day. The protocol called for the seven tubes to be removed from the cold incubator and the cells therein were to be processed in the FACS in order to separate the radioactive-dyed cells from the bystander non-radioactive non-dyed cells in each of the seven tubes. This action should have resulted in seven Helena tubes disposed of in the radioactive waste bin. Each of the original seven tubes should give rise to, ultimately, six 60 mm dishes to be cultured in the 37 degree incubator, three dishes to contain the radioactive-dyed cells plated for colonies and three dishes to contain the bystander, non-radioactive, non-dyed cells plated for colonies – 42 dishes in all.

By evening on Friday, March 30, the cold incubator should have been empty, there should have been seven empty Helena tubes in the radioactive trash and there should have been 42 60 mm tissue culture dishes in the 37 degree incubator. In fact, the cold incubator contained the holder with six Helena tubes that we had determined were both radioactive and contaminated. Furthermore, they were not removed until April 5. There were no Helena tubes in the radioactive trash. There were 42 dishes in the 37-degree incubator, and there was a Helena tube in the regular trash marked #7 in the same ink as the other six tubes. The contents of this tube were also found to be radioactive (and contaminated) and should not have been in that trash container.

On Wednesday, April 4, the dishes were to be washed, stained and counted for colonies. The results were unexpected and puzzling. The 21 dishes of cells that had been exposed to tritiated thymidine and the dye were all contaminated and could not be counted. There were, however, counts in the notebook in Howell's handwriting for 20 of the 21 non-radioactive, undyed cells (bystanders). Apparently, these dishes and the cells in them had not become contaminated.

The seven samples that were processed in the FACS on Friday cannot have been obtained from the seven Helena tube samples that had been in the 37 degree incubator since Tuesday, otherwise all of the 42 dishes would have been contaminated. The 20 (of 21) uncontaminated dishes most likely were set up using the uncontaminated cells that may have been obtained from Lenarczyk on Thursday evening.

Where did the 21 contaminated dishes come from? Tube number seven was the only tube that had been processed. The protocol also calls for radioactivity counts to be recorded from each of the original seven samples in the Helena tubes. Six of the seven were never processed and could not have been counted. However, the contents of number seven could have been diluted appropriately and counted to produce radioactive counts for the six other tubes. And, without thinking, the contents of number seven could also have been diluted to produce cells for the 21 dishes that would turn out to be contaminated, perhaps not realizing or forgetting about their likely contamination.

One last note regarding this experiment. Ironically, the terminal digits of the Coulter counts were not significantly different from random, and there were no averages found in the triplicate samples counted by Howell. Although there are plenty of questions to ask about this experiment, there is nothing in the statistical analysis to raise suspicions.

13. WHERE ARE THEY NOW?

If you don't have integrity, you have nothing
Henry Kravis

Anupam Bishayee, Ph.D.
The art of pleasing is the art of deception
Luc de Clapiers

Bishayee resigned his position in the Radiation Research Lab in July 2001 following the events described in Chapter 12. He spent a short time working in a laboratory in the Pharmacology Department then took a job as a Radiation Safety Officer in the Radiation Safety Department. He remained there until 2007 when he was able to obtain an Assistant Professor position in the Department of Pharmaceutical Sciences at a University in Ohio. He received an NIH grant and churned out papers, mostly reviews, at a high rate.

On August 6, 2015 Bishayee described his achievements on the web:

He had held academic positions in his field for twenty-five years. In the usual way, these would involve teaching, administration and research. He also was a charter member of the faculty in two pharmacy schools, rising to department chairman in two of them and assistant dean in one. His teaching expertise encompasses nine different pharmacy-related fields and he has researched dietary constituents of cancer-prevention and treatment-related plant products for 17 years. He has obtained private, public and governmental support for his research. He has written chapters in books published by high-level publishing houses. Most impressive, however, is his output listed on PubMed: as of May 5, 2016, he is credited with 110 articles of which 74 were published since leaving my institution and eight of which have been commented on in PubPeer. Thirty-three of his papers are classified as reviews.

Sometime around 2012, Jeffrey Beall, an academic librarian in Denver, CO, began surveying on-line journals and started a blog called Scholarly Open Access (http://scholarlyoa.com) on which he lists what he calls "potential, possible, or probable predatory scholarly open-access publishers" and "potential, possible, or probable predatory scholarly open-access journals". Serving as a journal editor, on an editorial board or being asked to review articles are among the hallmarks of academic success. Bishayee claimed to serve on the editorial board of 15 peer-reviewed journals. He listed himself as an Associate Editor of an international gastroenterology journal but was not even listed as a member of that editorial board. He was listed as associate editor of an on-line journal. He named 11 additional journals on which he claimed to be an editor. I was unable to find three of the journals he listed. He was not on the lists of editors of two of the journals on his list. Five of the remaining six journals are on Beall's lists. Since that time, he has pared down his list to four editorial boards, although he still claims to be on 15. Of the four, he remains on three, but still is not on one of the ones that he was not on last August. This happens to be one of the premier journals in his field.

Many individuals who have been sanctioned by the ORI in recent years have been found guilty of misrepresenting or manipulating figures and most especially photos of electrophoretic gels. Gel figures are easily altered using Adobe Photoshop® or some similar software. This is a form of scientific misconduct that is relatively easy to detect. Some of Bishayee's research papers have figures containing images of gels.

PubPeer is a website where virtually all papers in the scientific literature can be accessed for post-publication review. Many critiques involve analyses of images that appear to have been manipulated. The first of Bishayee's papers to be so exposed appeared in the *Journal of Carcinogenesis* in 2009.[42] Figure 3C in that article is made up of 6 photomicrographs in two rows. In my Figure 10, "a" is a photomicrograph of control tissue culture cells, "b" depicts cells incubated with drugs for 6 hours, in "c", the cells were similarly incubated for 12 hours, in "d", 24 hours, "e", 48 hours and "f" is another control. It is easy to see that c and d use the same photograph. However, the image in d has been slightly enlarged, cropped and smeared horizontally. An anonymous comment about this was posted on Pub Peer on December 1, 2013.

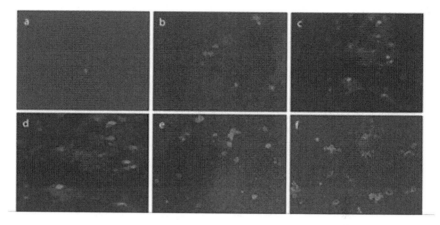

Figure 10. Taken from Figure 3 in Rabi T, Bishayee A.(2009).[42]

Questions also have been raised on PubPeer about gels in 7 other papers co-authored by Bishayee. Figures 11 - 16 are taken from some of Bishayee's publications since he left our medical school. Several of them may involve the use of a technique known as cloning defined by the Office of Research Integrity website[43] where the following statements appear:

- "The use of cloning or copying techniques to specifically create objects in an image that did not exist there originally is research misconduct (falsification, fabrication).
- "According to ORI investigator John Krueger, cloning and copying of data has frequently been used to falsify images. Because of the historical misuse of these tools, the undeclared use of cloning in a published image could lead to charges of research misconduct.
- "Examples of misconduct would include copying gel bands into an existing gel image to create a new result, and/or any other image "seamlessly" created from the combination of portions of two or more images."

Figures 11 through 16 are from 8 of Bishayee's *et al.* published papers. In the figures that follow, Beta-Actin (β-Actin), GAPDH and 18s RNA are loading controls, chemical species mixed in with the samples in each lane to correct for differences in loading the lanes.

C.

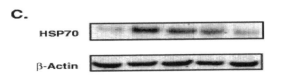

HSP70

β-Actin

Figure 11. Bishayee A, Waghray A, *et al.* (2010)[44], Figure 2C. HSP70: vertical background change and sharp demarcation between lanes 1 and 2, possibly between lanes 2 and 3 and between lanes 3 and 4. Suggest these lanes did not all come from the same gel, although the implication is that they did.

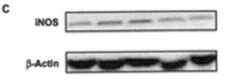

c

INOS

β-Actin

Figure 12. Bishayee A, Barnes KF, *et al.* (2010).[45] Figure 2C: INOS/Beta-actin: vertical displacement of actin (lane 4) not seen in INOS – Are these from the same gel? The implication is that they are.

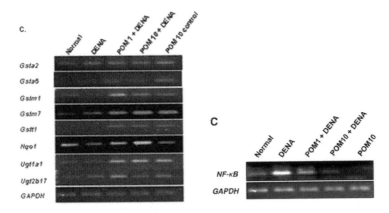

Figure 13. Left: Bishayee A, Bhatia D, *et al.* (2011).[46] Figure 3C. Right: Bishayee A, Thoppil RJ, *et al.* (2013).[47] Figure 5C. Note that the GAPDH panels are distinctive – suggest reuse of the same loading control (GAPDH) in 2 different studies. Each study – reported in different publications – should have its own loading control.

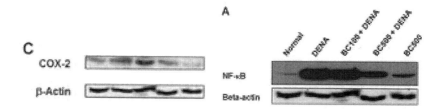

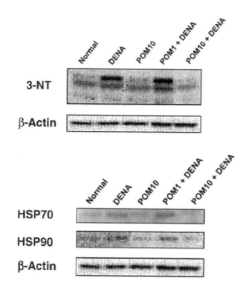

Figure 14. Bishayee A, Thoppil RJ, et al. (2013).[48] Figures 5C and 7A. The large vertical step between bands lanes 3 and 4 in beta-Actin is not seen in COX-2 and NF-kappaB. Suggest Beta-actins are not from the same gels.

Figure 15. Bishayee A, Thoppil RJ, *et al.* (2013)[47] Top: Figure 2C. 3NT vertical demarcation between lanes 2 and 3 and 3 and 4. Bottom. Figure 3D. HSP70: There is a vertical change of background between lanes 3 and 4; HSP90: there is a vertical change of background between lanes 2 and 3.

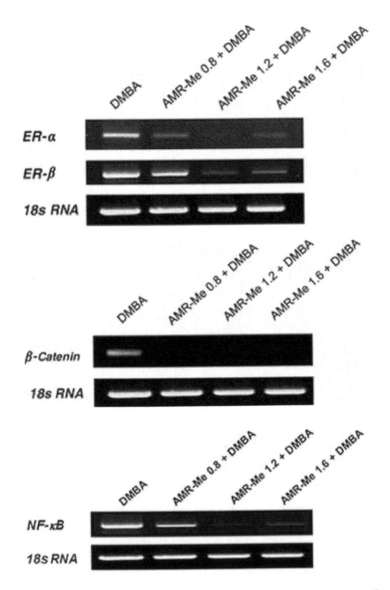

Figure 16. Upper 2 gels: Mandal A, Bhatia D *et al.* (2013).[49] Upper, Figure 3; lower, Figure 6. **Lower gel:** Mandal A, Bhatia D, *et al.*, (2014).[50] Figure 3D. Reuse of the same loading control (18S RNA) in 2 different studies.

Roger W Howell, Ph.D.

The intensity of the conviction that a hypothesis is true has no bearing on whether it is true or not

Peter Medawar

Howell was promoted to Professor in 2001, probably as a reward for being awarded the above NCI grant. He received the Loevinger-Berman Award from the Society of Nuclear Medicine "given in recognition of excellence pertaining to the field of internal dosimetry as it relates to nuclear medicine" in 2005. He was also awarded an Inventors prize by the UMDNJ several years ago and was elected Basic Science NJMS Faculty of the Year in 2009. He has also been Principal Investigator of an NIH challenge grant for "Protection Against Radiation-Induced Damage to Intestinal Nutrient Transport" for two years ending in February of 2011. He recently was awarded, along with Dr. Edouard Azzam, an NIH grant to study the bystander effect in radium-223 therapy, for three years with $421,612 for the first year.

14. ATTEMPTS TO PUBLISH

Justice will not be served until those who are unaffected are as outraged as those who care

Benjamin Franklin

After the *qui tam* case was filed in October 2003, and up to the time that it was closed, I was unable to discuss or reveal anything publically about the data that I was analyzing. My hands were tied with respect to publishing until October 18, 2010, when the District Judge filed his Opinion, and it became a dead letter when I lost the appeal on October 20, 2011.

The première science journals, *Science* and *Nature*, both have front sections devoted to various news articles. In both journals, as well as in newspapers like the *New York Times* and the *Washington Post,* there have been increasing numbers of reports of scientists gone bad. I mistakenly thought that, since there was an obvious interest in scientific misconduct, it would be an easy thing to publish our statistical methods of analysis in one or the other of these journals. I could not have been more wrong. In fact, we, Dr. Pitt and I, have been turned down, to date, by no less than 11 journals (see Table 11). Two of those rejections were appealed and failed. One journal, *Publications,* accepted our paper that focuses only on the two tritiated thymidine reports (papers 6 and 7, see above) and deals primarily with the radiation biology aspects of our analysis[2].

Our first submission was to the journal *Science* on June 15, 2011. Their response came on July 6 "Although your analysis is interesting, we felt that the scope and focus of your paper make it more appropriate for a more specialized journal". About a week later, we submitted a "Presubmission Inquiry" to *Nature,* which was rejected the next day for the reason that we proposed analyzing data that had not been in papers published in *Nature.* Still aiming high, we focused on *PLoS* (for *Public Library of Science*) *ONE,* a relatively new and increasingly popular on-line journal. Before submitting this time we sent it to the American Journal Editors who helped us shape up the language, punctuation and style. For this, we received a certificate suitable for framing, but, alas, *PLoS ONE* never sent the paper out for review, rejecting it in the Editorial Office in about three weeks. We appealed but to no avail.

In the original rejection, the *PLOS* Editor states "we feel that your manuscript does not address a specific research question or describe a research study *per se*. In addition, we are concerned that the analyses reported imply misconduct in relation to previous articles published elsewhere. In the light of this, and in accordance with accepted procedures in publishing ethics, we feel it is more appropriate for the journals that published original articles to pursue this matter." In appealing, we called attention to the guidelines listed on the COPE website. COPE (Committee on Publication Ethics) is a forum of publishers and editors that advises on the handling of cases of potential research and publication misconduct. The PLoS ONE Editor averred abidance by COPE's recommendations but placed the responsibility back on the editors of the journals that published the original articles.

The journal *Accountability in Research*, by its very name, seemed like the perfect journal to publish our article. I had previously sought advice from the Editor when looking for expert witnesses for the *qui tam* case. However, it seems the journal is more interested in portentous proclamations than in dealing with actual cases, so, again, the paper died in the editorial office.

Since half the papers published by Bishayee from the Radiation Research Lab were in *Radiation Research* the journal of the Radiation Research Society, of which I am a member, we decided to try there next. We submitted the paper and a cover letter of explanation to the Editor directly. He wasted no time in rejecting our efforts again. In his rejoinder, the Editor suggested that I could withdraw my name as co-author of one of the papers and that if I did so, Howell would be invited to submit a response. I consider this a last ditch possibility that, at the time of this writing, I have not acted on.

Next we submitted our paper to *Annals of Applied Research*, feeling confident that here it would be welcomed as this was the journal that had published the statistical analysis of chemotherapy studies at Duke University that have led to multiple retractions and several resignations[51]. It was rapidly rejected by the Associate Editor to whom it was assigned but he made some helpful comments which we took to heart, revised and resubmitted. It was again rejected by a different Associate Editor, but this time with permission to resubmit. Thus encouraged, we revised it again only to be definitively rejected. The critiques by the Associate Editor and the referee mainly had to do with format. The referee's comments were rather odd and his/her turns of phrase were "anodyne" (his/her word). We appealed to the Editor-in-Chief who politely declined to reconsider.

JOURNAL	DATE SUBMITTED	SCIENTIFIC REVIEW(S)	FINAL DECISION	DATE	EDITOR	COMMENTS
Science	6/14/11	No	Reject	7/6/11	Brooks Hanson, PhD	Low priority
Nature	7/13/11	No	Reject	7/15/11	Claudia Lupp, PhD	Not for us
PLOS ONE	1/24/12	No		2/10/12	Elizabeth Silva	Specific research question not addressed
Appeal	2/22/12	No	Reject	3/12/12	Iratxe Puebla, DPhil	
Accountability In Research	3/8/12	No	Reject	3/8/12	David B Resnick JD PhD	Not for us
Radiation Research	2/13/12	No	Refuse to consider	3/8/12	Marc Mendonca, PhD	Not for us
AoAS	3/13/12	+/-	Reject	3/16/12	Tilman Gneitling	Assoc Ed helpful
AoAS	9/13/12	+/-	Reject w resub	9/26/12	Susan Paddock	Form difficult to evaluate
AoAS resubmission	11/20/12	+/-	Reject	12/7/12	Susan Paddock	Not for us
FASEB-J	12/17/12	No	Reject	12/17/12	George Weissmann, MD	Form difficult to evaluate
ACTA ONCOL	2/20/13	Yes(2)*	Reject	3/6/13	Bengt Glimelius, Ph.D.	Not competitive
Appeal	3/9/13	Yes(5)**	Reject	5/2/13	Bengt Glimelius, PhD	Three reviewers supportive
Stats in Medicine	12/29/12	No	Reject	1/7/13	Dr Joel Greenhouse	Low priority
Micron	7/8/13	Call for retraction sent to Editorial Board			Dr Guy Cox	No action yet
The Amer Statistician	10/10/13	Yes (4)	Reject	3/18/14	Ronald Christensen, PhD	3 in favor, 1 opposed
Publications ***	2/28/14	Yes(6)	Accept	8/18/14	Dr R Grant Steen	All reviews favorable
BMC Medical Research Methodology	5/23/14	Yes(1)	Reject for all BMC Journals	9/22/14	Dr Giulia Mangiameli	Reviewer said yes
ScienceOpen Research	1/22/16	1 (Post Publication)	Accept	2/16/16	Stephanie Dawson	

* Reviews not sent ** 2 of 5 reviews not sent *** Not the same paper

Table 11. Disposition of journal submissions.

Bruce Ames, famous for the Ames test for mutagenesis/carcinogenesis, co-authored a series of exchanges in the *Life Sciences Forum* of the *FASEB Journal* in 2009, regarding massive data fabrication[52]. Following their lead, we submitted, as required, an Initial Inquiry: an abstract and cover letter, on December 17, 2012. Within hours, the submission was rejected. We then submitted to *Statistics in Medicine* on December 29, 2012. We were rejected after barely a week. The letter said

"Although the problem you are working on is interesting, the degree of methodological innovation is not at the level of development that would receive a high enough priority for publication in Statistics in Medicine".

Since one of the Howell-Bishayee papers we analyzed above, had been published in *Acta Oncologica* we decided to give that journal a try. The Editor wrote back that *Acta Oncologica* was not an appropriate journal, we asked that he reconsider and he graciously responded that he would. This was followed rather expeditiously by 3 rather thoughtful and encouraging reviews but the paper was still rejected. In any case, we were pleased to have finally had scientific reviews of our work.

Next, I decided to confront the Editor-in-Chief and the Editorial Board of *Micron* directly, elaborating on the statistical analysis of the data supporting the paper in the same manner as I have done in this book. Out of courtesy, copies of the letter were sent to Drs Howell, Bishayee, and Stephen Baker, Chairman of the Department of Radiology, the Deans for Research and Faculty Affairs at the New Jersey Medical School, Dr Virginia Barbour, the Chairman of COPE (Committee on Publication Ethics), a scientific and medical watchdog organization, and Ivan Oransky, co-blogger of the *Retraction Watch Blog*. This was followed on the Newark campus by a letter from the Dean of the New Jersey Medical School threatening to fire me if I did not cease and desist. Dr. Cox, the Editor, acknowledged receipt of the letter, promised to look into it, but now, more than two years later, no action has been taken.

Pitt was very interested in having the paper published in a statistics journal so we took many of the suggestions received from the *Acta Oncologica* reviewers, revised and submitted to *The American Statistician*. The paper was reviewed very favorably by the Associate Editor and two additional referees, but the Editor-in-Chief, it appears, really did not want to accept it (fear of law suits?) so he sent it to Dr. Terence Speed, a very brilliant Australian numbers person who was partly responsible for destroying the ORI's case against Thereza Imanishi-Kari who had been accused of data fabrication in the 1980's (see Chapter 16, below). In like manner, Speed destroyed our paper stating that we had put too much faith in statistical models. It had taken 5 months to reject our efforts and, by now, nearly 3 years had passed since our first attempt to publish in *Science.*

In December of 2013, we learned that there was to be a symposium-in-print to be published in the journal *Publications* entitled *Misconduct in Scientific Publishing* edited by R Grant Steen, who is well-known for his interest in scientific misconduct. The deadline for submissions was February 28, 2014. The paper that we submitted deals with only a portion of the data analyzed in this book: primarily the substance of papers 6 and 7 that deal with the bystander effect of tritiated thymidine. There were in all 6 reviews and numerous rewrites before the paper was finally accepted and published on September 1, 2014[2].

Meanwhile, we submitted a preprint to *BMC-Medical Research Methodology* and were encouraged to submit to that journal that we did in May 2014. It was reviewed quite favorably by, as far as we know, only one reviewer who recommended acceptance. Nevertheless, it was rejected in November of that year, along with a statement indicating it would not be welcomed by any other of the many BMC journals. That one reviewer turns out to be John Carlisle, who has contributed a chapter to this book.

On January 22, 2016, we submitted the paper to *ScienceOpen Research,* an on-line journal that ascribes to post-publication review[2]. The paper was accepted in May and thus far (June, 2016) has been reviewed once. The review is very thoughtful and detailed. The reviewer gave it 3.5 stars out of 5 overall. For importance and validity, it received 4 stars each but for level of comprehensibility, only two. Obviously, it needs more work. But at least it is out there and others can see it. An earlier version is also posted on the pre-print server *ArXiv*[2].

Our quest has not gone unnoticed. I was featured as one of three whistle-blowers in an article in *Nature* in November 2013: http://www.nature.com/news/Research ethics: 3 ways to blow the whistle-1.14226. *The Scientist* published an Opinion Piece by me in February 2014: Opinion: Reducing Whistleblower Risk | The Scientist Magazine. Moreover, I was interviewed by Ralph Nader on his Radio Show on April 14, 2015. The podcast can be heard by going to www.ralphnaderradiohour.com.

To publish this book, I chose LULU, a self-publisher that offers additional assistance for formatting and editing. I paid about $2000 for the program. Not unsurprising, it took me far longer than anticipated to get my analyses off the ground. In fact, it was over a year before I sent them an initial draft. And then I heard nothing from them for several months. When I did finally hear, it was to tell me that they could not publish the book as is. Here were their concerns: my letter from ORI director Wright could not be published because it was marked confidential. But I am not publishing the letter from Wright, merely summarizing it. Judge Cavanaugh's decision is off limits even though he is a federal judge whose decision is freely available on the web. Furthermore, his decision is summarized not quoted. I was exhorted to disguise all the players by using a pen name for myself, false names for everyone else in the book, false names for all businesses and educational establishments, change the locations, obtain notarized permissions from all parties discussed. I tried to comply but in the end, I just simply could not. I have done my best to state only that which is true and that I can back up with documents. I have stated my opinions and my intention is to make it clear that these are my opinions. I contacted LULU and told my contact that I could simply not comply with their requirements. Much to my surprise, they have refunded almost all of my money and I have to hand it to them for doing that. The book is now being published by HillTree Farm Press and printed by Create Space, an Amazon Company that offers on-line directions for formatting but cannot assist me further because I have too many figures and tables. I am, therefore, pretty much on my own and I apologize for any irregularities in the text and in formatting. I have also used Grammarly© to spot my many errors in syntax.

15. A LOOK IN THE MIRROR

I sent my Soul through the Invisible,
Some letter of that After-life to spell:
And by and by my Soul return'd to me,
And answer'd: 'I Myself am Heav'n and Hell'

Omar Khayyam

One of my goals is to encourage scientists to monitor continuously data that is generated in their labs in order to stop potential misconduct before it even has a chance to start. What better place to start than in my own laboratory. Over the years, I have had a number of technicians, post-doctoral fellows and students. Much of my research has involved the plating of colonies on tissue culture dishes. This started with my graduate school studies where I investigated the effects of ultraviolet and visible light on the ability of the alga, *Euglena gracilis*, to restore the green pigment, chlorophyll, to its bleached chloroplasts[53]. The dishes in these experiments were 100 mm in diameter and the medium in which the colonies grew was semi-solid agar. Later on in my career, I studied the effects of ionizing radiation (gamma- and X-rays) and various wave lengths of ultraviolet light on survival of malignant melanoma cells that varied in their pigment content. In this case, the colonies expanded in 35 mm dishes in liquid tissue culture medium. Our samples were always plated in triplicate – that seems to be the *modus operandi* for experiments in which colony forming ability is involved. I have notebooks full of data eminently suitable for analysis using the tests described and employed in earlier chapters.

I extracted over 1000 triples from experiments performed by 6 members of my group. Table 12 summarizes the results of Test 1 where the numbers of triples with the exact mean, K, can be compared to the expected numbers, N ± std, to determine the corresponding Z-values and the probabilities of K or greater. K is less than N for investigators A, C, D, E and F. Pitt designed the model to give the subject whose data was under scrutiny the benefit of the doubt, so to speak – therefore, the model overestimates the expected number of exact means. K is more than N for investigator B only. In the interest of openness, my own *Euglena* colony counts are recorded under Investigator E.

INVESTIGATOR	# TRIPLES	K=# W MEAN	N=# EXPECTED	STD	Z-VALUE	P≥K
A	222	33	37.4	5.5	-0.88	0.81
B	132	34	24.6	4.5	2.0	0.026
C	75	8	14.7	3.4	-2.1	0.99
D	329	30	61.3	7.0	-4.5	1.00
E	199	9	21.4	4.4	-3.0	1.00
F	90	11	18.6	3.8	-2.1	0.99

Table 12. Exact Means In The Triplicate Colony Counts Of 6 Investigators In The Hill Lab Over A Period Of 40 Years

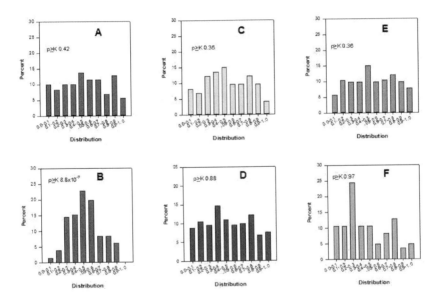

Figure 17. Mid-ratio Distributions From Colony Counts of Investigators in the Hill Lab. The probabilities of K or more colony counts in the 0.4 to 0.6 range are shown on the graphs. Number of triples: A, 219; B, 132; C, 74; D, 328; E, 194; F, 88.

Figure 17 shows the mid-ratio distributions for colony counts of the same investigators. K, in this case, is the number of triples in which the mid-ratios are in the 0.4-0.6 range, and N is the corresponding number expected in that range. The $p \geq K$ values shown on the graphs are the corresponding probabilities. All are greater than or equal to 0.35 except for investigator B.

Cells in my lab were observed microscopically and were counted using a hemocytometer. As a result, there are no Coulter counts to evaluate. The terminal digit distributions of the colony counts are shown in Figure 18. The p-values are 0.24 or greater except for investigators A and B. A's skewed distribution is dominated by a preference for terminating with zero. Such rounding of hand-counted colonies to the nearest decile would not be good science but would have little impact on interpretation of the results. Can the same be said for B's terminal digit distributions? S/he appears to have a preference for 5's. This could just be sloppy work, but taken in the context of B's other probabilities, $p \geq K$ of 8.8×10^{-7} for mid-ratios and 0.026 for the number of exact means in the triples, one cannot help but wonder if B's terminal digit distributions of 1.1×10^{-9} are a reflection of some data manipulation. The paper that featured these data was published in 1997 and has been cited 15 times, most recently in 2008.

The mid-ratio distribution for F's colonies is clearly bizarre, but does not reflect any tendency to focus the triples around the means. There may be some other explanation than data fabrication. At that time in my lab, plating for colonies did not employ disposable pipet tips such as were used for each dish in the Radiation Research lab. Those triplicate colony numbers were independent. The pipets used for plating in my lab had a capacity of 1.0 milliliter. The dishes in the triads each received 0.2 milliliters of cell suspension from a single pipet. Therefore, the counts in the 3 dishes in each triple were not independent. The cells in the pipet tended to settle and plating had to been done rapidly, otherwise the three dishes would not receive the same number of cells. I speculate that the uneven distribution of mid-ratios in F's profile is the result of a technical error and not the result of any intent to defraud. This is further supported by F's terminal digit distribution which is consistent with random or uniform. If this holds for F, should it not hold also for B? B's results are suspicious on all 3 fronts: exact means in triples, mid-ratios and terminal digit distribution.

The analysis of the numbers generated in my lab is very instructive. Had I but had the statistical tools that are now available, I could have encouraged A to refrain from influencing the colony counts. I would have corrected F's plating technique, and I would have kept a very close eye on B's results, to the point of checking his/her data points myself. Were I to be doing these experiments in my lab today, I would have an automatic colony counter with a hard copy printout for recording the colony counts.

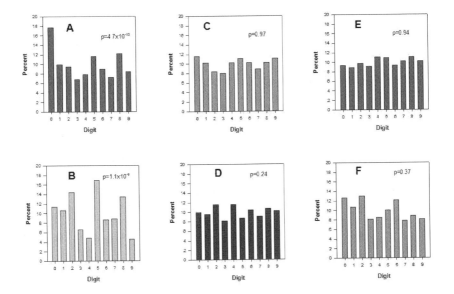

Figure 18. Terminal Digits of Colony Counts of Various Investigators. The probabilities that the distributions are uniform or random are shown for each graph. Numbers of counts: A, 666; B, 396; C, 225; D, 987; E, 597; F, 270.

16. STATISTICS AS A FORENSIC TOOL

The first principle is that you must not fool yourself - and you are the easiest person to fool

Richard Feynman

Perhaps the easiest type of data falsification to detect is image manipulation – using Photoshop® to insert bands or lanes into photographs of electrophoresis gels, flipping images to elude detection of inserted bands. The website PubPeer allows subscribers – who may choose to remain anonymous – to critique essentially any paper that has a Digital Object Identifier, DOI, a form of registration. In like manner, PubMed allows comments from registrants to PubMed Commons following the specific citations. Submissions to PubPeer consist of critiques, discussions, reviews and, inevitably, notations about and images of suspected data manipulation. PubMed Commons lists some but not all comments that have appeared in PubPeer. Recent entries to PubPeer are listed on the website's introductory page and are visible at log on. I sampled the first 30 so listed on July 24, 2015. Of these, 15 involved image manipulations and only 5 referred to statistical criticisms of one form or another. Clearly, it is the low-hanging fruit - the images - that are getting the most attention.

Falsification and manipulation of numbers is certainly not new and has probably been going on since numbers were invented. In modern times, one of the first and foremost of spin doctors may well be Gregor Mendel, the father of modern genetics.[54] The chi-square test was introduced by Karl Pearson in 1900, 16 years after Mendel's death. It did not take long after this for the statistician, Ronald A Fisher, to use the new test to analyze Mendel's numbers which seemed to be too good and to calculate that their chance of occurrence in dozens of experiments was on the order of one in ten thousand or less. Mendel probably had a good idea, after a time, of what he wanted to prove. Can we hold it against him that he was more picky and less objective than he should have been? On the other hand, did he secretly think that no one would find out and that he would get away with it? Was this scientific misconduct? Or just a form of exaggeration? Does this tarnish his integrity?

In more recent times, one highly publicized case that has had a great impact on the way academic institutions and the government deal with scientific misconduct is that of Thereza Imanishi-Kari, a junior colleague of David Baltimore, a Nobel prize winner, eminent scientist and academician[55]. At the time the scandal broke in the mid-1980's, Imanishi-Kari was a junior faculty member at MIT studying the genetics of the immune system in mice. A post-doctoral fellow in her laboratory, Margot O'Toole, had been unable to repeat some key experiments and believed that earlier results had been fabricated. Her cause was quickly espoused by two scientists at the NIH, Ned Feder and Walter Stewart, and by John D. Dingell, US Representative from Michigan. Imanishi-Kari was found guilty of serious scientific misconduct and was barred from receiving federal funds for a period of 10 years. She appealed and was later completely exonerated by the Appeals Board of the Department of Health and Human Services, a one-sided board only available to defendants and not to whistle-blowers.

But had she falsified data? A website, www.conductinscience.com, posted by Charles W. McCutchen, PhD, by now a retired physicist at the NIH, presents compelling statistical arguments that she may have. Imanishi-Kari's experiments involved counting of samples of mouse cell extracts that had been tagged with gamma ray emitting radioactive iodine. Some of the radioactive counts had been hand-copied from tapes – bearing some resemblance to the method used in the Radiation Research Lab to record Coulter counts. McCutcheon presents a histogram on his website of the frequencies of various gamma ray counts ranging from 210 to 480 from one of Imanishi-Kari's experiments. The bar graph of the counts is said to be spikey and quite different from similar data recorded directly onto the tape of a gamma ray counter without human intervention. Imanishi-Kari admitted that, in some cases, the units digit had been rounded to the nearest 10 and that she had been careless when transcribing the data. One aspect noted by McCutcheon that makes the data suspicious, however, is the periodicity of her counts. The patterns repeat at 100 count intervals. James E. Mosimann, the statistician for the ORI, analyzed the terminal digits of Imanishi-Kari's data for uniformity using the chi squared test and found them to be significantly non-uniform leading him to believe that they had been fabricated. Terence Speed, an expert witness for Imanishi-Kari, without mentioning it, combined the so-called bins of counts by 3's but did not point out that this eliminated the spikiness that had concerned Mosimann. The Appeals Board was persuaded more by Speed's arguments than by Mosimann's. McCutcheon calculates that the chance that Imanishi-Kari's numbers were as spikey or spikier by bad luck is 1 in 10^{32}. Speed also killed Pitt's and my submission to *The American Statistician* (see Chapter 14 above).

The ORI was burned by the Imanishi-Kari case and it has led them to tread lightly ever since. This is eminently clear in my own case. They had in their hands at the time of their investigation numerical data from Bishayee and from me. The number of samples was grossly inadequate and they could easily have asked for more but did not – cf above, Table 1 - in which the terminal digit Chi squared p for uniformity is 0.07 for the other investigators (Controls) compared to 10^{-95} for Bishayee. Alan Price who was in charge of the ORI investigation in my case stated confidently in a phone conversation revealed in the Discovery documents that he doubted it would be possible to find controls. Had he but asked, the University could have furnished over 2000 individual control Coulter counts.

In order to get an idea of how well the ORI has been doing over the years, I compared data presented in three of their annual reports: 1994, the first year of reporting, 2002, and 2012, the most recent year for a report. In 1994, the ORI responded to 185 "queries", while in 2002, there were 191 and in 2012, 423 "allegations". In 1994, 44 cases were closed, 67 carried over to 1995 and in 6, misconduct was found. In 2002, 32 cases were closed, 50 carried over and in 13, falsification and fabrication were found. In 2012, 35 cases were closed, 79 carried over and misconduct was found in 14. The change in 18 years is modest considering the fact that over this span of years there has been about a 10-fold increase in retractions of which about half are estimated to be due to some kind of fraud[56]. Is the ORI keeping up or is it falling behind the trend? Or does it look the other way?

In 2005, Martinson *et al.* published a Commentary in *Nature* reporting a survey with about a 50% response rate from 3247 scientists. About 40% of the responders admitted to engaging in serious misconduct and/or questionable practices[57]. Granted, little of these would rise to the level of serious misconduct, but it does reflect a fundamental attitude of *laissez-faire* among scientists. In a more recent publication, Fang, Steen and Casadevall calculate that misconduct accounts for well over half of retracted studies listed in PubMed as of May 2012[58].

When it comes to image manipulation, a good set of eyes is really all it takes. When numbers are fudged, it takes intuition and a good set of tools for measuring. P-values of 0.05 may be making things too hard on miscreants, but where to draw the line? One chance in one hundred? One chance in one thousand? This is something that needs to be decided among the *cognoscenti*. Different tests are necessary to measure different ways of manipulating the data. Other reasons for discrepancies must be considered and explored. Some of these matters are dealt with by Al-Marzouki, *et al.* in an article published in the British Medical Journal in 2005[59]. Akhtar-Danesh and Dehghan-Kooshkghazi, in a study comparing real and made-up data sets, observed that high correlation coefficients were a likely indication of fabricated data[60]. Uri Simonsohn was able to detect data fabrication by two researchers from statistical analysis of their reported means and standard deviations alone[61], leading him to argue for posting of raw data, a requirement that should be endorsed by all scientists interested in keeping the record straight. Hudes, *et al.* reported finding unusual clustering of coefficients of variation in 84 articles from 3 investigators in a Biochemistry department of a university in India. For their controls, Hudes, *et al.* searched PubMed to find 26 similar studies by others that failed to show similar clustering. The original article was published in The FASEB Journal and was additionally interesting as the "accused" authors had the opportunity to rebut the Hudes, *et al.* article, to which Hudes, *et al.* again responded[62].   Such interchanges seem eminently fair. The accused should always be given an opportunity to respond.

The specialty of Anesthesiology seems to have been particularly prone to problems of misconduct. Joachim Boldt, a German anesthesiologist, has been accused of fabricating data and other unethical conduct in some 90 publications and at one point held the record for the highest number of retractions in the Retraction Watch blog (www.retractionwatch.com). Scott Reuben, an anesthesiologist at Baystate Medical Center in Springfield, MA, spent 6 months in prison as a result of his misconduct.   He fabricated data in some 22 articles and was caught as a result of statistical analysis that determined his data violated the Newcomb

Benford Law that involves the digit frequencies of leftmost digits, as opposed to rightmost digits in the studies that are reported in this book. Yoshitaka Fujii, another anesthesiologist, currently holds the record for the most retractions, on the order of 170. He, too, was caught by statistics. And his misdeeds also led to a lively exchange in the journal *Anaesthesia* by the Editors, the whistle-blower -- none other than John Carlisle -- who has graciously joined me in contributing to this book, Hudes, *et al.* and Fujii himself. This exchange was recently reviewed in the *Nautilus* magazine[63]. Carlisle compared Fujii's published distributions of some 28 variables with expectations of chance and found p values ranging from 0.04 to less than 1 in 10^{33} [64].

Rutgers professor Robert Trivers along with Brian Palestis and Darine Zaatari published a book, *Anatomy of a Fraud*[65], in 2009 aimed at revealing data fabrication by a former post-doctoral fellow in Trivers' lab that had been published in a paper in *Nature*[66]. The paper concluded that there are "strong positive associations between symmetry and dancing ability, and these associations were stronger in men than in women". In the book, the authors claim that post-doctoral fellow William Brown had altered data by removing good dancers from the asymmetric group and poor dancers from the symmetric group in order to achieve statistical significance between the groups. They calculated, summing over all the parameters that were measured, that there was a probability of 1 in 10^{10} that Brown's results could have been due to chance. Trivers case has some parallels to mine – not just that we are both Rutgers professors. One of the co-authors of the paper in question has refused to admit the deception and *Nature* dragged its feet for 8 years before allowing the paper to be retracted. The wishy-washy retraction mentions nothing about wrong-doing, much to Trivers' disgust. Since then, Trivers, an icon in the field of human behavior, has received shoddy treatment from Rutgers, far worse than the threat that I received from my Dean.

There may be as many statistical methods for detecting fraud as there are stars in the sky. In this discussion, I have tried to mention a few. An additional study that should not be forgotten is that of Baggerly and Coombes published several years ago in the *Annals of Applied Statistics*[67]. Their paper demonstrates that simple errors, like switching columns on Excel sheets, can lead to misleading results that impact on therapeutic choices for specific cancer patients. Their study resulted in the firing of Anil Potti, a medical oncologist at Duke University, 11 law suits and the retraction or correction of 18 papers (www.retractionwatch.com). Potti, not to be outdone, has resurfaced as a medical oncologist at a cancer center in Grand Forks, North Dakota, with two and a half stars out of five in evaluations from 14 patients.

Up to this point, journals have taken a back seat when it comes to retractions. Bornmann, et al.[68] surveyed 46 research studies to determine editorial grounds for rejection or acceptance. Nine criteria were prominent but none were related to falsification or fabrication – this in spite of the findings of Fang, *et al.*[58]. Truth, it would seem, did not play a role. Retraction Watch has just recently reported that 35% of the world's top-ranking science journals don't have a retraction policy and this is considered to be "an improvement". 94% of those that have a policy do allow the editors to retract articles without authors' consent. They also point out that some scientists seem to mistakenly believe that only authors can retract a paper. This is important since I was told by the Editor of *Radiation Research* that it would be "illegal" for him to initiate retractions. Perhaps now he can be persuaded to change his mind.

17. WHO CARES?

Be leery of silence. It doesn't mean you won the argument. Often people are just busy reloading their guns
Shannon L. Adler

In the spring of 2012, I set up a website (www.helenezhill.com) where I tell my story and make available most of the relevant documents. Since May 30 of that year, there have been over 5400 visitors. More specific website data are only available since November, 2015. Of the visitors since then, 33% have spent more than 30 seconds on the site, and as many as 10 spent 1 to 2 hours. Visitors come from all six continents and 69 different countries. In the US, most visitors come from New Jersey followed by California. During the early years, data that no longer shows on the website, there was considerable activity from around Rootstown, OH, the home of Northeastern Ohio Universities where Bishayee held his first academic appointment. From February to November of 2015, there were 19 visitors from Los Angeles County where he was Chairman of a department in a pharmacy school, 18 in the region of his next appointment, but none from around Miami where he is now a department Chairman in another pharmacy school.

Searching on the web (June, 2016) brings up Bishayee's name associated with the article in *Nature* (www.nature.com/news/research-ethics-3-ways-to-blow-the-whistle-1.14226) about my struggles, my Opinion article in *The Scientist* (http://www.the-scientist.com/?articles.view/articleNo/39139/title/Opinion--Reducing-Whistleblower-Risk/), and the District Court judgment (www.vernialaw.com/FCA Documents/DCT/2010/US ex rel Hill v......UNITED STATES DISTRICT COURT DISTRICT OF NEW JERSEY). The Larkin School of Pharmacy, his current employer, was apparently undeterred by these reports. Howell's scientific accomplishments are quite prominent on a web search and his struggles with justice have all but disappeared. Science has forgiven him.

After I blew the whistle in 2001, I became *persona non grata* in the Division of Radiation Research and have been shunned by its members since then. My office moved to another part of the building next door to the office of the Senior Associate Dean for

Research. After the article about me and two other whistle-blowers came out in *Nature*, I posted it on my door. This Dean was also copied on the letter that I wrote to the Editor of *Micron* that contains most of the analysis of paper 8 (see above). In spite of the fact that he must know of my activities, and research misconduct must surely be something that would be of concern to him and to his office, he has never asked me anything about it, even though he passes by my door every day when he goes to the men's room. We did once have a short exchange and all I can remember is that he brushed it off with "Oh that". In similar fashion, I sent email to the wife of Rutgers University president, an ethicist, requesting to work with her at making the system of dealing with whistle-blowers and scientific integrity more equitable and fair. I received a return receipt that my email to her had been read but I never received a reply. For that matter, only one person out of all the many passing by my door has stopped in to comment and congratulate me for my efforts.

The Associate Dean for Faculty Affairs was also copied on the *Micron* letter. At that time, she chaired the Department of Microbiology and Molecular Genetics in which I held a secondary appointment. We have crossed paths in the hallways, but she, too, passes me by without any acknowledgment. Virginia Barbour, Chairman of the Committee on Publication Ethics (COPE) was informed about my case and our attempts to publish. And she was copied on the letter to *Micron*. She responded to my email promising to review the situation but I never heard from her again.

My efforts to confront the Radiation Research Society have brought the greatest frustration. The editor of the official journal of that society, *Radiation Research,* has dug his heels in and is not the least bit interested in pursuing retraction of any of the four papers analyzed above. I spoke to him last year at the Annual Meeting of the Society and he told me it would be illegal for him to initiate retractions, although a number of journals have done so. It is pretty clear that Howell, himself, refuses to admit that the data have been fabricated, so it is unlikely that he will agree to retracting any of the four papers in *Radiation Research,* analyzed above, unless he is ordered to do so. I also have spoken to two former presidents of that Society. One expressed great interest and sympathy but has done nothing. The other collaborates on grants with members of the Radiation Research Division at the New

Jersey Medical School. His research is intertwined with theirs. I met with him last year and he confirmed his unwillingness to have anything to do to help me even though I know that he has useful information. A former friend, he now treats me like dirt.

The scientific community turns a blind eye on scientific misconduct. Scientists are only interested when it happens in their lab or when they, themselves, are caught. The fellowship of whistle blowers support each other to some extent, but there is little to gain by preaching to the choir.

Do people in authority do their homework? Do members of NIH Study Sections who are instrumental in awarding grants look into the backgrounds of prospective Principal Investigators? Do they, for example, perform internet searches on them? And if they find questionable behavior, why do they award grants to such people when they could easily award young investigators who are just getting a start? Why do medical and pharmacy schools appoint department heads with shady pasts that are easily traced and even have evoked comments questioning their integrity on PubPeer and PubMed?

It is all about the money. But

You're still left alone with yourself in the end.
Billy Idol

AFTERWORD

Corn cannot expect justice from a court composed of chickens

African proverb

In my attempts to report what I believed to be misconduct, I failed at every round. Perhaps that was all to the good. My journey makes clear what needs to change in order to make the system fair, to prevent and, once it occurs, to deal with allegations of scientific misconduct. Academic institutions have too large a stake in the outcomes, so their role should be minimized. They could start the process by determining whether allegations have any validity but after that, they should step aside.

A new paradigm for truth in science:

1. Each state should establish a Board of Scientific Examiners that will adjudicate each case. Science can be very complicated so there must be *ad hoc* members with expertise in the field in question but with no personal relationships with either the whistle-blower(s) or the accused. States have Boards of Medical, Pharmacy, Nursing and Veterinary Examiners. Why not a Board for Scientists?

2. All raw data must be made publically available unless there is some over-riding reason, such as national security, to keep it confidential

This includes numerical data such as are analyzed here. For gels, photographs of entire gels should be presented to the reviewers to prevent mixing results of different studies

3. Scientists should be obliged to report failed replication attempts to the journals that published the results, to their academic institutions and to their funding agencies

4. Scientists should be free to critique the works of others without fear of reprisals or law suits, as long as their criticism is made in good faith

5. All misconduct hearings involving state and federally funded research should be open to the public

6. All reports should be open to the relevant parties and to the public

7. Regarding formal accusations, both the complainant(s) and the respondent(s) should have the right to appeal to some higher level body such as the appropriate Office of an Inspector General

8. Journals should take a more active role in retracting papers that contain false information

9. Journals acting in good faith should be protected from law suits

10. There is a need for a journal that publishes scientific controversies where conflicting data can be presented and disagreements can be heard without fear of retribution

11. Statistical analysis of numerical data needs to come in to its own as a valid method for the detection of scientific fraud

12. Humans are fallible. Data should be evaluated and recorded by tamper-proof instruments whenever possible

13. Data analysis should be blinded, names should be anonymized whenever possible

Beware:

We only see what we look for, we only look for what we know

Francis D. Moore, M.D.
paraphrasing Johann Wolfgang von Goethe

And now, a question: Should scientific misconduct be considered to be a crime? If it is a crime to falsify financial reports, then why is it not a crime to falsify scientific and medical reports? If it is a civil offense then should the miscreants, Institutions and perpetrators, be required to repay the funds in question and receive no more funds until this is done?

SUPPLEMENT: ADDITIONAL NUMERICAL ANALYSIS

By John B Carlisle

Statistics is the grammar of science.
Karl Pearson

Introduction

On the 30th July 2014 I received an email from Professor Oliver Kuss, asking me to review an article submitted by Helene Hill and Joel Pitt to *BMC Medical Research Methodology*. I had experience analysing summary data, such as mean (SD), from randomised controlled trials to identify data distributions inconsistent with random allocation. However, I had not had the opportunity to analyze the distribution of separate measurements of observational data.

The trigger to the analyses by Hill and Pitt was the suspicion that particular data were fabricated. I thought that the focus of the analysis on fabrication might have alienated the editors of the *BMC* and other journals. I thought that a more general exploration of the data might reveal unusual distributions that in turn would lead to competing explanations only one of which might be data fabrication. Unusual data distributions require explanation. Data distributions that are inconsistent with distributions from similar experiments or that are incompatible with an expected distribution are worrisome. A study sample that has a distribution that is inconsistent with similar studies may be unrepresentative of the experiment being tested. The greater the disparity between the distribution of one sample and samples from similar experiments, the greater should be the interrogation of those data. One would logically conclude that the results of an experiment would be wrong if the data that generated those results deviated from expected distributions, or from distributions observed in similar experiments. The greater the deviation, the greater should be the circumspection with which one uses deviant data. Extreme differences in data distributions would preclude drawing safe conclusions from results of experiments. That is, it is not necessary to prove fabrication to conclude that data are too unsafe to publish unless those data have been validated.

The data supplied by Hill and Pitt consisted of rows of three columns, with a number in each row's column. What characteristics could one examine in these rows? One could analyze the digits as if they did not represent quantities. One could count the number of digits contained in each number, how many digits are unique in each number in the triplicate, and how many are repeated. One could analyze the total number of digits in a triplicate that ranged from 3 to 15. One could analyze the digits as ordered, but again ignore the quantities that they represent: for instance '3' comes before '6' in the order '0 to 9'. One could analyze the digits in each number as representing a quantity. This is how one usually looks at numbers, for instance, '123' is more than the sequence, it is the number 'one hundred and twenty-three'. One could look at the magnitude of the numbers in a triplicate, read from left to right. For instance, if 'a', 'b' and 'c' represent the smallest, middle and largest numbers, the sequence in each row could be: 'abc', 'acb', 'bac', 'bca', 'cab' or 'cba' (ignoring ties). One could analyze the values of digits in particular positions in each number, for instance, the first or last numeral. One could analyze the quantitative relationship between the numbers in a row.

All of these characteristics of a row have little power to determine data authenticity if the rows are analyzed independently. I analyzed data with the available categorising criteria: the type of data coded by the numbers (colony counts or Coulter counts); the experimental set (usually consisting of 10 rows); the date the rows were recorded (predominantly the same as the experimental set); the identity of the scientist recording the data. My null hypothesis was that the distribution of data in each category for each criterion was the same.

I analyzed the sequence of numbers in a row. I assumed that the sequence of counts would be randomly ordered. Deviations might be due to chance or some process that affected the numerical size, for instance increasing Coulter counts of a cell suspension that became more concentrated. Another explanation would be that the investigator recorded a preliminary, randomly-ordered sequence, which was then ordered on entry into the official record. I also analyzed the terminal digits of each number. I assumed that the rate of terminal digits from '0' to '9' would be uniformly distributed. Deviations might be due to chance, a restricted range of small numbers (for instance between 2 and 6), or an abnormal counter on a Coulter counter that favored particular digits. Another explanation would be an investigator 'rounding' numbers up or down to reach a preferred terminal digit. I also analyzed the value of the numbers in a triplicate to determine whether their distribution was consistent across categories and whether their distribution was consistent with some parametric distributions.

Methods

I analyzed triplicate data generated by a single laboratory between 15th April 1992 and 21st May 2005, as described elsewhere by Hill. I used Pearson's chi-squared and Fisher exact tests to analyze the rates of ordered numbers in a triplicate and the rates of terminal digits. I conducted pairwise posthoc tests, adjusted with the method of Benjamini and Yekutieli. I generated p-values for each triplicate through Monte Carlo simulations of the following distributions: Poisson; negative binomial; Weibull. I used Kolmogorov-Smirnov tests of the distribution of p-values against the expected uniform distribution. I used Kruskal-Wallis rank sum and ANOVA tests for the interaction of p-values with people who recorded the data: in the event of a significant result I conducted pairwise Wilcoxon rank sum tests (p-value adjusted with Benjamini and Yekutieli) and pairwise Games-Howell test after ANOVA. Independent p-values were combined with Stouffer's method for each data source. Analyses were conducted in R.

Results

They were all out of step but Jim
                                        Irving Berlin

I analyzed 2992 complete colony triads and 2646 complete Coulter count triads.

Triad sequences and terminal digits of numbers

Table JC1 is the rates of ordered triad sequences for each investigator, and Table JC3 lists the posthoc pairwise p-values. Table JC2 is the rates of terminal digits for every triad number, and Table JC4 lists the posthoc pairwise p-values. Q provided most data, so subtotals of all other authors (TOTAL − Q) are provided for comparison in Tables JC1 and JC2.

Investigator	Cou/col	'abc'	'acb'	'bac'	'bca'	'cab'	'cba'	Total	Chi sq	P value
Q	Coulter	351	211	202	250	286	384	1684	>31	1.11x10⁻¹⁹
	Colony	397	131	138	120	307	236	1329	>31	3.86x10⁻⁶⁰
	Total	748	342	340	370	593	620	3013	>31	2.68x10⁻⁶³
G	Coulter	16	14	20	18	16	13	97	2.1	0.84
	Colony	17	1	2	2	2	2	26	>31	1.74x10⁻⁸
	Total	33	15	22	20	18	15	123	11.0	0.051
A	Coulter	-	-	-	-	-	-			
	Colony	36	32	29	49	26	41	213	10.1	0.073
	Total	36	32	29	49	26	41	213	10.1	0.073
C	Coulter	-	-	-	-	-	-			
	Colony	17	16	11	6	12	11	73	6.5	0.262
	Total	17	16	11	6	12	11	73	6.5	0.262
H	Coulter	3	1	10	9	11	14	48	15.5	8.43x10⁻³
	Colony	4	7	8	6	6	7	38	1.4	0.92
	Total	7	8	18	15	17	21	86	11.1	0.049
I	Coulter	5	1	2	3	4	9	24	10.0	0.075
	Colony	48	48	44	46	44	50	280	0.55	0.99
	Total	53	49	46	49	48	59	304	2.1	0.83
J	Coulter	34	82	56	89	61	72	394	30.0	1.48x10⁻⁵
	Colony	49	35	37	26	30	41	218	9.2	0.10
	Total	83	117	93	115	91	113	612	10.6	0.061
B	Coulter	-	-	-	-	-	-			
	Colony	20	22	20	31	26	13	132	8.5	0.13
	Total	20	22	20	31	26	13	132	8.5	0.13
K	Coulter	31	39	26	34	34	43	207	5.1	0.40
	Colony	7	13	5	13	17	15	70	9.2	0.10
	Total	38	52	31	47	51	58	277	10.7	0.057
L	Coulter	12	5	7	9	12	14	59	6.0	0.31
	Colony	10	8	10	7	11	4	50	4.0	0.55
	Total	22	13	17	16	23	18	109	3.9	0.56
M	Coulter	4	2	3	3	1	7	20	6.4	0.27
	Colony	1	0	1	1	2	2	7	2.4	0.79
	Total	5	2	4	4	3	9	27	6.5	0.26
N	Coulter	5	9	8	10	10	10	52	2.2	0.82
	Colony	2	0	2	2	2	4	11	4.8	0.44
	Total	7	9	9	12	12	14	63	3.2	0.67
O	Coulter	-	-	-	-	-	-			

								Total	Chi sq	P value
	Colony	3	1	3	0	2	4	13	5.0	0.42
	Total	3	1	3	0	2	4	13	5.0	0.42
D	Coulter	-	-	-	-	-	-			
	Colony	115	46	49	45	24	34	313	>31	8.09×10^{-20}
	Total	115	46	49	45	24	34	313	>31	8.09×10^{-20}
F	Coulter	-	-	-	-	-	-			
	Colony	45	16	5	10	6	6	88	>31	5.30×10^{-16}
	Total	45	16	5	10	6	6	88	>31	5.30×10^{-16}
Total	Coulter	461	364	334	425	435	566	2585	>31	3.97×10^{-15}
	Colony	791	398	383	395	543	483	2993	>31	8.62×10^{-51}
	Total	1252	762	717	820	978	1049	5578	>31	7.40×10^{-46}
Total-Q	Coulter	110	153	132	175	149	182	901	23.9	2.31×10^{-4}
	Colony	394	267	245	275	236	247	1664	>31	3.31×10^{-12}
	Total	504	420	377	450	385	429	2565	25.2	1.27×10^{-4}

Table JC1 Triads categorised by the order in which the numbers were recorded in columns from left to right: 'a' the largest number; 'b' the middle number; 'c' the smallest number.

*Fewer than 2992 colony triads and 2646 Coulter count triads were categorized as the same number occurred two or three times in some triads. For colony vs Coulter distribution [†]p = 3.99×10^{-17} and [‡]p = 1.71×10^{-10}.

Investigator	Cou/Col	0	1	2	3	4	5	6	7	8	9	Total	Chi sq	P value
Q	Coulter	475	613	736	416	335	732	363	425	372	718	5185	467	7.1×10^{-95}
	Colony	564	324	463	313	290	478	336	408	383	526	4085	201	2.3×10^{-38}
	Total	1039	937	1199	729	625	1210	699	833	755	1244	9270	526	1.2×10^{-107}
G	Coulter	25	28	31	25	41	29	32	30	33	36	310	7	0.64
	Colony	11	8	8	10	11	7	6	13	6	7	87	6	0.74
	Total	36	36	39	35	52	36	38	43	39	43	397	6	0.74
A	Coulter	-	-	-	-	-	-	-	-	-	-	-		
	Colony	118	66	63	45	52	77	60	48	81	56	666	62	4.7×10^{-10}
	Total	118	66	63	45	52	77	60	48	81	56	666	62	4.7×10^{-10}
C	Coulter	-	-	-	-	-	-	-	-	-	-	-		
	Colony	26	23	19	18	23	25	23	20	23	25	225	3	0.97
	Total	26	23	19	18	23	25	23	20	23	25	225	3	0.97
H	Coulter	12	14	13	12	19	18	11	21	21	12	153	9	.040
	Colony	16	9	16	16	12	10	16	11	16	12	134	6	0.78
	Total	28	23	29	28	31	28	27	32	37	24	287	5	0.83
I	Coulter	7	6	11	8	16	15	7	12	9	4	95	15	0.103
	Colony	78	78	85	81	94	101	85	83	94	85	864	6	0.74
	Total	85	84	96	89	110	116	92	95	103	89	959	11	0.30
J	Coulter	124	155	137	124	132	117	137	140	143	130	1339	8	0.52
	Colony	77	84	87	69	73	67	68	69	84	69	747	7	0.62
	Total	201	239	224	193	205	184	205	209	227	199	2086	12	0.21
B	Coulter	-	-	-	-	-	-	-	-	-	-	-		
	Colony	45	42	57	26	19	67	34	35	53	18	396	61	1.1×10^{-9}
	Total	45	42	57	26	19	67	34	35	53	18	396	61	1.1×10^{-9}
K	Coulter	59	59	62	55	68	59	79	41	82	76	640	22	9.4×10^{-3}
	Colony	26	30	29	22	17	24	15	25	24	28	240	9	0.44
	Total	85	89	91	77	85	83	94	66	106	104	880	14	0.11
L	Coulter	13	23	17	17	18	21	12	20	19	20	180	6	0.75
	Colony	17	16	11	12	26	16	20	18	13	25	174	13	0.15
	Total	30	39	28	29	44	37	32	38	32	45	354	10	0.39
M	Coulter	6	4	8	7	5	7	8	4	8	3	60	5	0.80
	Colony	1	0	5	5	4	2	3	5	3	2	30	9	0.41
	Total	7	4	13	12	9	9	11	9	11	5	90	9	0.47
N	Coulter	15	22	16	11	19	24	12	15	16	15	165	9	0.43
	Colony	2	3	3	5	1	2	3	4	2	5	30	5	0.80
	Total	17	25	19	16	20	26	15	19	18	20	195	6	0.75
O	Coulter	-	-	-	-	-	-	-	-	-	-	-		
	Colony	4	2	2	8	4	3	7	6	2	4	42	10	0.36
	Total	4	2	2	8	4	3	7	6	2	4	42	10	0.36
D	Coulter	-	-	-	-	-	-	-	-	-	-	-		
	Colony	98	95	114	80	114	86	103	90	106	101	987	12	0.24
	Total	98	95	114	80	114	86	103	90	106	101	987	12	0.24
F	Coulter	-	-	-	-	-	-	-	-	-	-	-		
	Colony	34	29	35	22	23	27	33	21	24	22	270	10	0.37
	Total	34	29	35	22	23	27	33	21	24	22	270	10	0.37
Total	Coulter	736	924	1031	675	653	1022	661	708	703	1014	8127	296	1.7×10^{-58}
	Colony	1117	809	997	732	763	992	812	856	914	985	8977	153	2.2×10^{-28}
	Total	1853	1733	2028	1407	1416	2014	1473	1564	1617	1999	17104	329	2.0×10^{-65}
Total-Q	Coulter	261	311	295	259	318	290	298	283	331	296	2942	16	0.07
	Colony	553	485	534	419	473	514	476	448	531	459	4892	34	1.1×10^{-4}
	Total	814	796	829	678	791	804	774	731	862	755	7834	31	1.1×10^{-4}

Table JC2 Rate of terminal digits in the triad numbers.

Table JC3 Adjusted p-values for pairwise comparisons of triad sequences, calculated from Table JC1.

	Q	G	H	I	J	K	L	M	N	O	A	B	F	C
G	0.5													
H	4×10^{-2}	0.2												
I	2×10^{-2}	1	1											
J	$<10^{-5}$	7×10^{-2}	1.0	1										
K	6×10^{-4}	7×10^{-2}	0.9	1	1									
L	1	1	1	1	1	1								
M	1	1	1	1	1	1	1							
N	1	1	1	1	1	1	1	1						
O	1	1	1	1	1	1	1	1	1					
A	2×10^{-4}	1	0.8	1	1	1	1	1	1	1				
B	6×10^{-4}	1	0.4	1	1	1.0	1	0.5	1	1	1			
F	$<10^{-5}$	2×10^{-2}	$<10^{-5}$	$<10^{-5}$	$<10^{-5}$	$<10^{-5}$	4×10^{-4}	2×10^{-2}	1×10^{-4}	0.1	$<10^{-5}$	$<10^{-5}$		
C	0.9	1	0.2	1	1	1	1	1	1	1	0.9	1.0	5×10^{-2}	
D	$<10^{-5}$	1	$<10^{-5}$	$<10^{-5}$	$<10^{-5}$	$<10^{-5}$	1×10^{-2}	0.3	6×10^{-3}	1	2×10^{-4}	3×10^{-4}	0.8	0.4

Table JC4 Adjusted p-values for pairwise comparisons of terminal digits, calculated from Table JC2.

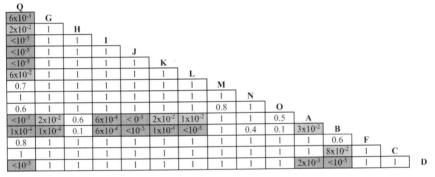

	Q	G	H	I	J	K	L	M	N	O	A	B	F	C
G	6×10^{-3}													
H	2×10^{-2}	1												
I	$<10^{-5}$	1	1											
J	$<10^{-5}$	1	1	1										
K	$<10^{-5}$	1	1	1	1									
L	6×10^{-2}	1	1	1	1	1								
M	0.7	1	1	1	1	1	1							
N	1	1	1	1	1	1	1	1						
O	0.6	1	1	1	1	1	1	0.8	1					
A	$<10^{-5}$	2×10^{-2}	0.6	6×10^{-4}	$<10^{-5}$	2×10^{-2}	1×10^{-2}	1	1	0.5				
B	1×10^{-4}	1×10^{-4}	0.1	6×10^{-4}	$<10^{-5}$	1×10^{-4}	$<10^{-5}$	1	0.4	0.1	3×10^{-2}			
F	0.8	1	1	1	1	1	1	1	1	1	1	0.6		
C	1	1	1	1	1	1	1	1	1	1	1	8×10^{-2}	1	
D	$<10^{-5}$	1	1	1	1	1	1	1	1	1	2×10^{-3}	$<10^{-5}$	1	1

Triad distributions

The distribution of triads for Coulter counts were explored separately from the distribution of triads for colony counts.

Table JC5 Colony triads tested against Poisson and negative binomial distributions.

Author	n	Poisson distribution			Negative binomial distribution		
		Mean	SD	p-value	Mean	SD	p-value
Expected		*0.500*	*0.289*	*1*	*0.50*	*0.289*	*1*
Q	1361	0.258	0.229	$< 10^{-16}$	0.246	0.219	$< 10^{-16}$
G	29	0.521	0.298	0.79	0.502	0.290	0.92
A	222	0.590	0.304	2.9×10^{-5}	0.545	0.283	2.1×10^{-2}
C	75	0.611	0.281	9.3×10^{-3}	0.560	0.254	0.085
H	45	0.459	0.260	0.26	0.427	0.236	0.057
I	288	0.557	0.305	2.0×10^{-3}	0.506	0.280	0.30
J	249	0.512	0.291	0.71	0.483	0.274	0.35
B	132	0.442	0.259	2.3×10^{-2}	0.416	0.243	3.3×10^{-4}
K	80	0.485	0.292	0.67	0.462	0.280	0.49
L	58	0.509	0.269	0.80	0.485	0.257	0.80
M	10	0.382	0.279	0.24	0.372	0.273	0.21
N	10	0.479	0.290	0.87	0.460	0.280	0.65
O	14	0.687	0.290	8.8×10^{-3}	0.647	0.268	2.9×10^{-2}
D	329	0.674	0.285	$< 10^{-16}$	0.602	0.266	1.1×10^{-8}
F	90	0.664	0.293	1.5×10^{-6}	0.601	0.269	2.5×10^{-5}

Colony triad distributions

Table JC5 lists the results of comparing the distribution of triad numbers against Poisson distributions and negative binomial distributions, which the triads most approximated. The binomial and Weibull distributions were less consistent with the triad distributions, and their results are not presented, except one author (see below).

Table JC6 a) Adjusted p-values (Games-Howell method after ANOVA) for pairwise comparisons of colony Poisson p-values.

Q	G	H	I	J	K	L	M	N	O	A	B	F	C	D
6×10^{-4}	1	H												
$<10^{-16}$	1	0.6	I											
1×10^{-43}	1	1	0.9	J										
1×10^{-7}	1	1	0.8	1	K									
3×10^{-7}	1	1	1	1	1	L								
1.0	1	1	0.8	1	1	1	M							
0.6	1	1	1	1	1	1	1	N						
5×10^{-3}	0.9	0.4	0.9	0.7	0.6	0.7	0.4	0.9	O					
1×10^{-13}	1	0.2	1	0.2	0.3	0.8	0.6	1	1	A				
8×10^{-11}	1	1	7×10^{-3}	0.5	1	1	1	0.4	0.2	2×10^{-4}	B			
4×10^{-10}	0.6	5×10^{-3}	0.1	2×10^{-3}	6×10^{-3}	6×10^{-2}	0.3	0.8	1	0.8	1×10^{-6}	F		
$<10^{-16}$	1	0.2	1.0	0.4	0.3	0.7	0.5	1	1	1	3×10^{-3}	1	C	
$<10^{-16}$	0.4	3×10^{-4}	1×10^{-4}	8×10^{-9}	7×10^{-5}	4×10^{-3}	0.2	0.7	1	0.1	6×10^{-13}	1	0.9	D

Table JC6 b) Adjusted p-values (Benjamini-Yekutieli method after Kruskal-Wallis) for Wilcoxon pairwise comparisons of colony Poisson p-values.

Q	G	H	I	J	K	L	M	N	O	A	B	F	C	D
1×10^{-4}	G													
2×10^{-6}	1	H												
$<10^{-16}$	1	0.4	I											
$<10^{-16}$	1	1	0.7	J										
6×10^{-11}	1	1	0.6	1	K									
2×10^{-10}	1	1	1	1	1	L								
0.9	1	1	0.6	1	1	1	M							
0.2	1	1	1	1	1	1	1	N						
1×10^{-4}	0.6	0.2	1	0.3	0.3	0.4	0.3	0.6	O					
$<10^{-16}$	1	0.1	1	0.1	0.1	0.4	0.4	1	1	A				
6×10^{-14}	1	1	3×10^{-3}	0.3	1	1	1	1	0.1	1×10^{-4}	B			
$<10^{-16}$	0.3	2×10^{-3}	0.1	6×10^{-4}	2×10^{-3}	2×10^{-2}	0.1	0.4	1	0.6	3×10^{-7}	F		
$<10^{-16}$	1	0.1	1	0.1	0.1	0.3	0.3	1	1	1	7×10^{-4}	1	C	
$<10^{-16}$	0.1	1×10^{-4}	6×10^{-5}	2×10^{-9}	1×10^{-5}	6×10^{-4}	0.1	0.3	1	3×10^{-2}	4×10^{-13}	1	0.4	D

Table JC6 is a comparison of one author with another for distributions of colony p-values generated by testing against Poisson distributions, using: a), posthoc parametric pairwise comparisons; b), posthoc non-parametric pairwise comparisons. Table JC7 is the same, but for p-values generated by testing against negative binomial distributions.

Table JC7 a) Adjusted p-values (Games-Howell method after ANOVA) for pairwise comparisons of colony negative binomial p-values.

Q	G	H	I	J	K	L	M	N	O	A	B	F	C	D
4×10^{-3}	G													
6×10^{-4}	1	H												
$<10^{-16}$	1	0.8	I											
1×10^{-13}	1	1	1	J										
2×10^{-7}	1	1	1	1	K									
3×10^{-7}	1	1	1	1	1	L								
1	1	1	0.9	1	1	1	M							
0.6	1	1	1	1	1	0.1	1	N						
5×10^{-3}	1	0.4	0.8	0.7	0.6	0.8	0.5	0.9	O					
3×10^{-13}	1	0.2	1	0.5	0.6	1	0.8	1	1	A				
3×10^{-10}	1	1	5×10^{-2}	0.4	1	0.9	1	1	0.2	6×10^{-4}	B			
4×10^{-10}	0.9	8×10^{-3}	0.1	1×10^{-2}	4×10^{-2}	0.2	0.4	0.9	1	0.9	8×10^{-6}	F		
$<10^{-16}$	1	0.3	1	0.7	0.7	0.7	1	1	1	1	2×10^{-2}	1	C	
$<10^{-16}$	0.9	2×10^{-3}	2×10^{-5}	2×10^{-6}	7×10^{-3}	0.1	0.5	0.9	1	0.6	4×10^{-10}	1	1	D

Table JC7 b) Adjusted p-values (Benjamini-Yekutieli method after Kruskal-Wallis) for Wilcoxon pairwise comparisons of colony negative binomial p-values.

Q	G	H	I	J	K	L	M	N	O	A	B	F	C	D
8×10^{-6}	G													
3×10^{-6}	1	H												
$<10^{-16}$	1	0.9	I											
$<10^{-16}$	1	1	1	J										
2×10^{-10}	1	1	1	1	K									
3×10^{-10}	1	1	1	1	1	L								
0.9	1	1	1	1	1	1	M							
0.2	1	1	1	1	1	1	1	N						
1×10^{-4}	1	0.1	0.8	0.4	0.5	0.5	0.3	0.9	O					
$<10^{-16}$	1	0.1	1	0.2	0.4	1	0.7	1	1	A				
2×10^{-13}	1	1	3×10^{-2}	0.3	1	0.9	1	1	4×10^{-2}	1×10^{-4}	B			
$<10^{-16}$	0.8	3×10^{-3}	0.1	4×10^{-3}	2×10^{-2}	0.1	0.3	1	1	0.6	4×10^{-4}	F		
$<10^{-16}$	1	0.1	1	0.6	0.5	1	0.6	1	1	1	3×10^{-3}	1	C	
$<10^{-16}$	0.8	7×10^{-4}	5×10^{-4}	1×10^{-6}	3×10^{-3}	3×10^{-2}	0.9	0.2	1	3×10^{-2}	4×10^{-10}	1	1	D

Coulter triad distributions

Table JC8 lists the results of comparing the distribution of triad numbers against Poisson distributions and negative binomial distributions, which the triads most approximated. The binomial and Weibull distributions were less consistent with the triad distributions, and their results are not presented, except for one author (see below).

Table JC8 Coulter triads tested against Poisson and negative binomial distributions.

Author	n	Poisson distribution			Negative binomial distribution		
		Mean	SD	p-value	Mean	SD	p-value
Expected		*0.500*	*0.289*	*1*	*0.50*	*0.289*	*1*
Q	1717	0.364	0.262	$< 10^{-16}$	0.327	0.237	$< 10^{-16}$
G	102	0.521	0.265	0.29	0.455	0.246	1.4×10^{-2}
H	51	0.545	0.285	0.43	0.481	0.265	0.76
I	25	0.560	0.406	2.1×10^{-3}	0.463	0.360	0.087
J	405	0.554	0.307	8.0×10^{-4}	0.464	0.278	2.8×10^{-2}
K	211	0.610	0.317	4.2×10^{-7}	0.491	0.287	0.28
L	60	0.522	0.301	0.46	0.472	0.276	0.36
M	20	0.419	0.307	0.27	0.350	0.276	6.0×10^{-3}
N	55	0.518	0.312	0.42	0.480	0.296	0.68

Figure JC1 Testing of the distributions of triad numbers against Poisson and negative binomial distributions, respectively; A. Colonies; B. Coulters

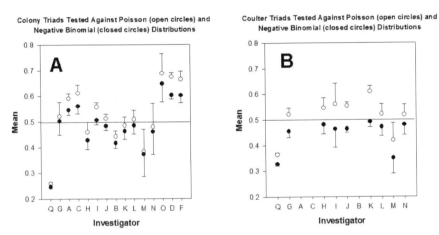

Table JC9 is a comparison of one author with another for distributions of p-values generated by testing against Poisson distributions, using: a), posthoc parametric pairwise comparisons; b), posthoc non-parametric pairwise comparisons. Table JC10 is the same, but for p-values generated by testing against negative binomial distributions.

Table JC9 a) Adjusted p-values (Games-Howell method after ANOVA) for pairwise comparisons of Coulter Poisson p-values.

Q	G	H	I	J	K	L	M	N
2×10^{-6}	G							
1×10^{-3}	1	H						
0.3	1	1	I					
4×10^{-10}	1	1	1	J				
1×10^{-13}	0.2	0.9	1	0.5	K			
5×10^{-3}	1	1	1	1	0.6	L		
1	0.9	0.8	0.9	0.6	0.2	0.9	M	
2×10^{-2}	1	1	1	1	0.6	1	1	N

Table JC9 b) Adjusted p-values (Benjamini-Yekutieli method after Kruskal-Wallis) for Wilcoxon pairwise comparisons of Coulter Poisson p-values.

Q	G	H	I	J	K	L	M	N
6×10^{-7}	G							
3×10^{-4}	1	H						
0.4	1	1	I					
$< 10^{-16}$	1	1	1	J				
$< 10^{-16}$	0.1	1	1	0.4	K			
3×10^{-3}	1	1	1	1	0.4	L		
1	1	1	1	1	0.4	1	M	
2×10^{-2}	1	1	1	1	0.4	1	1	N

Table JC10 a) Adjusted p-values (Games-Howell method after ANOVA) for pairwise comparisons of Coulter negative binomial p-values.

Q	G	H	I	J	K	L	M	N
3×10^{-5}	G							
4×10^{-3}	1	H						
0.6	1	1	I					
4×10^{-10}	1	1	1	J				
1×10^{-12}	1.0	1	1	1.0	K			
4×10^{-3}	1	1	1	1	1	L		
1	0.8	0.7	1	0.7	0.5	1	M	
8×10^{-3}	1	1	1	1	1	1	1	N

Table JC10 b) Adjusted p-values (Benjamini-Yekutieli method after Kruskal-Wallis) for Wilcoxon pairwise comparisons of Coulter negative binomial p-values.

Q	G	H	I	J	K	L	M	N
4×10^{-6}	G							
1×10^{-3}	1	H						
1	1	1	I					
$< 10^{-16}$	1	1	1	J				
9×10^{-14}	1	1	1	1	K			
2×10^{-3}	1	1	1	1	1	L		
1	1.0	1	1	1	1	1	M	
4×10^{-3}	1	1	1	1	1	1	1	N

Comparisons of Q versus other authors

Q contributed most data that were different from those of other authors. Figure JC2 illustrates the distribution of p-values for triad colony counts generated by comparison with Poisson distributions and negative binomial distributions. These distributions are presented for all authors (Fig. JC2a and JC2b) and Q versus others (Fig. JC2c and JC2d). Figure JC3 illustrates the same comparisons for triad Coulter counts.

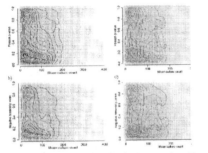

Figure JC2 The distribution of the mean of triplicate culture colony counts vs. p-values (dots), generated by one million Monte Carlo simulations of each triplicate, using: Poisson distributions (upper left and right); negative binomial distributions (lower left and right). Upper figures are results of all authors; right hand figures: separate data for Q and others. The shaded area is the kernel probability density estimate, overlaid by density decile contour lines. The vertical distribution of p-values would be homogeneous if triads followed Poisson distributions: upper graphs, or negative binomial distributions: lower graphs.

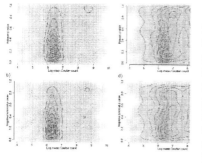

Figure JC3 The distribution of the natural logarithm of the mean triplicate Coulter count vs. p-values (dots), generated by one million Monte Carlo simulations of each triplicate, using: top graphs, Poisson distributions; bottom graphs, negative binomial distributions. Left hand figures are results of all authors, right hand figures, separate data for Q and others. The shaded area is the kernel probability density estimate, overlaid by density decile contour lines. The vertical distribution of p-values would be homogeneous if triads followed Poisson distributions: upper graphs, or negative binomial distributions: lower graphs.

Figures JC4 and JC5 depict the distribution of cumulative p values for Q versus other authors: triad colony counts generated by a Poisson distribution (Fig. JC4); triad Coulter counts, generated by a negative binomial distribution (Fig. JC5). Figure JC6 below is the cumulative p-value for each data source.

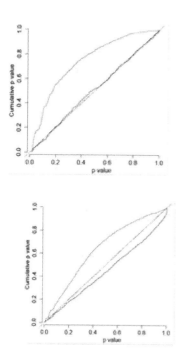

Figure JC4 Cumulative Poisson p-values for colony triplicate counts by Q (grey) vs. other investigators (black). The distribution of p-values by Q was different from expected (dashed black diagonal), $p < 10^{-16}$, while the distribution of p-values was as expected for other investigators, $p = 0.48$.

Figure JC5 Cumulative negative binomial p-values for triad Coulter counts by Q (grey) vs. other investigators (black). The distributions of p-values by both Q and the other investigators were different from expected (dashed black diagonal), $p < 10^{-16}$ and $p = 2 \times 10^{-8}$, respectively.

Summary of comparisons of observed data distributions versus parametric data distributions

Table JC11 summarizes the analyses of the triads. Figure JC6 is the cumulative p-value with and without that for triad sequence.

Table JC11 Summary of p-values for each data source for three triad characteristics. The distribution of colony triads approximated the Poisson distribution while the distribution of the Coulter triads approximated the negative binomial distribution, so these are the p-values reported.

Dataset Triad characteristic Distribution	Colony Distribution Poisson	Coulter Distribution Negative binomial	Combined Terminal digit Uniform	Combined Sequence Uniform
Q	$< 10^{-16}$	$< 10^{-16}$	2.9×10^{-50}	1.4×10^{-30}
D	$< 10^{-16}$	–	0.75	2.5×10^{-7}
F	1.5×10^{-6}	–	0.85	3.1×10^{-5}
A	2.9×10^{-5}	–	1.5×10^{-3}	0.43
B	2.3×10^{-2}	–	2.5×10^{-4}	0.50
O	8.8×10^{-3}	2.9×10^{-2}	0.86	0.64
M	0.24	6.0×10^{-3}	0.85	0.72
J	0.71	2.8×10^{-2}	0.74	0.37
I	1.9×10^{-2}	8.7×10^{-2}	0.82	0.96
K	0.67	0.28	0.60	0.34
G	0.79	1.4×10^{-2}	0.97	0.44
C	9.3×10^{-3}	–	1	0.63
H	0.26	0.76	0.98	0.28
L	0.80	0.36	0.86	0.84
N	0.87	0.68	0.97	0.90

Figure JC6 The cumulative p-value for each data source: with (black) and without (white) the p-value for the sequence in Table JC11. Note the logarithmic scale i.e. each mark from right to left on the horizontal axis is 100 million times less likely.

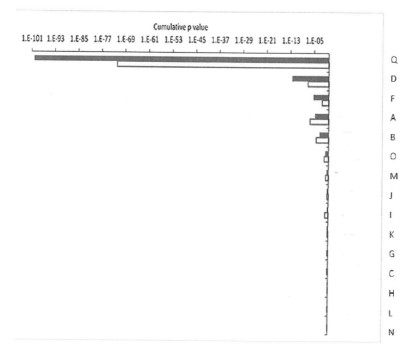

Discussion

Q was the single source that provided most data. Therefore s/he had the most power to generate small p-values when the observed distribution of data for triad sequence, terminal digits and distribution deviated from the parametric distributions (uniform, Poisson or negative binomial). However, the extent of deviation from parametric distributions was most for Q, which also deviated from the observed distributions of other data sources.

The distribution of colony triads provides the most convincing evidence that there was something wrong with the data of Q. The pooled data from other sources were consistent with Poisson distributions, but Q's data were extraordinary, as illustrated in Figure JC6. The distribution of Coulter triads were different for Q when compared to data pooled from other sources, although neither were consistent with Poisson, negative binomial or Weibull distributions. The distribution of Q's Coulter counts in each triad were less varied than expected for these distributions while their distribution was more varied than expected for data pooled from other sources. Malfunctions in the Coulter counter could account for deviations of observed versus expected distributions, but one would have to conclude that the malfunction was different in Q's experiments than other experiments. Discrepancies from a uniform distribution for terminal digits provide the next level of evidence for experimenters biasing their results. The range of numbers was sufficiently large to expect a uniform distribution of terminal digits 0-9. Q and two other data sources exhibited distributions of terminal digits consistent with the experimenters biasing counts. The weakest evidence for experimenters modifying their results was the sequence in which the numbers within a triad were reported: the sequence does not alter the results of the experiment. However, deviations do indicate active manipulation of results even if the consequences are benign.

Figure JC6 summarizes how cautious one should be accepting the results of experiments. The discrepancy of Q's data dwarfed the doubt pooled for other data sources. It is so extreme that one would conclude that the data are invalid. Studies based upon Q's data might be retracted on this evidence alone, even more so when one considers the concern that already existed for the propriety of these experiments.

18. LIST OF ABBREVIATIONS

CCRI   Campus Committee on Research Integrity

cGray   Centi-Gray, a unit of radiation measurement

COPE   Committee on Publication Ethics

DHHS   US Department of Health and Human Services

DMSO   Dimethylsulfoxide

DOI   Digital Object Identifier

FACS   Fluorescence Activated Cell Sorter

MEA   2-mercaptoethanolamine (cysteamine)

LED   Light Emitting Diode (Coulter Counter display of cell counts)

NCI   National Cancer Institute

NIH   National Institutes of Health

ORI   Office of Research Integrity

OSF   Open Science Framework

Std or sd   Standard deviation

USPHS   Unites States Public Health Service

Lab refers to the Radiation Research Lab

Raw data from Discovery documents are listed in the Appendix of the color version of this book. The Discovery PDF files containing scans from the Lab notebooks of the protocols and raw data are also available to the public, as are the Excel files derived therefrom and the Pitt Analyzer© for calculating results from Tests 1, 2 and 3. Go to https://osf.io/. Search Helene Z Hill.

REFERENCES

[1] Puck, T.T., Marcus, P.I. and Cieciura, S.J. 1956. Growth characteristics of colonies from single HeLa cells with and without a "feeder" layer. J. Exp. Med. 103: 273-284.

[2] Pitt, J.H. and Hill, H.Z. 20 November, 2013. Statistical detection of potentially fabricated numerical data. arXiv:1311.5517; HZ Hill, JH Pitt Failure to replicate: A sign of scientific misconduct? Publications 2: 71-82; doi:10.3390/publications2030071; JH Pitt, HZ Hill. Statistical analysis of numerical preclinical radiobiological data. ScienceOpen Research DOI: 10.14293/S2199-1006.1.SOR-STAT.AFHTWC.v1

[3] Mosimann, J. E., J. E. Dahlberg, et al. 2002. Terminal digits and the examination of questioned data. Accountability in Research 9: 75-92; Mosimann, J. E., D. V. Wiseman, et al. (1995). "Data fabrication: Can people generate random digits?" *Accountability in Research* 4: 31-55.

[4] Bishayee A, Hill HZ, Stein D, Rao DV, Howell RW. (2001) Free-radical-initiated and gap junction-mediated bystander effect due to nonuniform distribution of incorporated radioactivity in a three-dimensional tissue culture model. Radiation Research 155:335-344.

[5] Bishayee A, Rao DV, Howell RW. (1999) Evidence for pronounced bystander effects caused by nonuniform distributions of radioactivity using a novel three-dimensional tissue culture model. Radiation Research 152:88-97.

[6] Hall, E.J. 2003. The Bystander Effect. 85: 31-35.

[7] Nagasawa, H.; Little, J. B., Induction of sister chromatid exchanges by extremely low doses of alpha-particles. Cancer Res 1992, 52 (22), 6394-6.

[8] Shao, C.; Furusawa, Y.; Aoki, M.; Ando, K., Role of Gap Junctional Intercellular Communication in Radiation-Induced Bystander Effects in Human Fibroblasts. Radiation Research 2003, 160 (3), 318-323.

[9] Hu B, Han W, Wu L, Feng H, Liu X, Zhang L, Xu A, Hei TK, Yu Z. In situ visualization of DSBs to assess the extranuclear/extracellular effects induced by low-dose alpha-particle irradiation. Radiat Res. 2005 Sep; 164(3):286-91.

[10] Vines, A. M., F. M. Lyng, B. McClean, C. Seymour, C. E. Mothersill. 2008. Bystander signal production and response are independent processes which are cell line dependent. *Int. J. Radiat. Biol.* 84: 83-90

[11] Chan, P. C.; Lisco, E.; Lisco, H.; Adelstein, S. J., The radiotoxicity of iodine-125 in mammalian cells II. A comparative study on cell survival and cytogenetic

responses to 125IUdR, 131IUdR, and 3HTdR. *Radiat Res* 1976, 67 (2), 332-43.

[12] Bagley, C.G. Six red flags for suspect work. *Nature* 2013, 497, 433-434.

[13] Hall, E.J. and Giaccia, A.J. 2011 Radiobiology for the Radiologist. Lippincott, Williams and Wilkins 7th Ed 2011

[14] Tobey, R.A., E.C. Anderson, D.F. Petersen 1967 The effect of thymidine on the duration of G1 in Chinese hamster cells. J. Cell. Biol. 35: 53-39.

[15] Ehmann, U. K.; Williams, J. R.; Nagle, W. A.; Brown, J. A.; Belli, J. A.; Lett, J. T., Perturbations in cell cycle progression from radioactive DNA precursors. Nature 1975, 258 (5536), 633-6.

[16] Hoy, C. A.; Lewis, E. D.; Schimke, R. T., Perturbation of DNA replication and cell cycle progression by commonly used [3H]thymidine labeling protocols. Mol Cell Biol 1990, 10 (4), 1584-92.

[17] Hu, V. W.; Black, G. E.; Torres-Duarte, A.; Abramson, F. P., 3H-thymidine is a defective tool with which to measure rates of DNA synthesis. Faseb J 2002, 16 (11), 1456-7.

[18] Pollack, A.; Bagwell, C. B.; Irvin, G. L., 3rd, Radiation from tritiated thymidine perturbs the cell cycle progression of stimulated lymphocytes. Science 1979, 203 (4384), 1025-7.

[19] Bjursell, G.; Reichard, P., Effects of thymidine on deoxyribonucleoside triphosphate pools and deoxyribonucleic acid synthesis in Chinese hamster ovary cells. J Biol Chem 1973, 248 (11), 3904-9.

[20] Fox RM, Tripp EH, Tattersall MH: Mechanism of deoxycytidine rescue of thymidine toxicity in human T-leukemic lymphocytes. Cancer Res 1980, 40(5):1718-1721.

[21] Hiramoto, K.; Narahara, K.; Kimoto, H., Synchronization culture of amniotic fluid cells using excess thymidine block followed by deoxycytidine release and its application to high-resolution banding analysis of chromosomes. Jinrui Idengaku Zasshi 1990, 35 (2), 195-206.

[22] Morris, N. R.; Fischer, G. A., Studies concerning inhibition of the synthesis of deoxycytidine by phosphorylated derivatives of thymidine. Biochim Biophys Acta 1960, 42, 183-4.

[23] Wheater, R. F.; Roberts, S. H., An improved lymphocyte culture technique: deoxycytidine release of a thymidine block and use of a constant humidity chamber for slide making. J Med Genet 1987, 24 (2), 113-4.

[24] Burki, H. J.; Okada, S., Killing of cultured mammalian cells by radioactive decay of tritiated thymidine at -196 degrees C. Radiat Res 1970, 41 (2), 409-24.

[25] Bedford, J. S.; Mitchell, J. B.; Griggs, H. G.; Bender, M. A., Cell killing by gamma rays and beta particles from tritiated water and incorporated tritiated thymidine. Radiat Res 1975, 63 (3), 531-43.

[26] Burki, H. J.; Koch, C.; Wolff, S., Molecular suicide studies of 125I and 3H disintegration in the DNA of Chinese hamster cells. Curr Top Radiat Res Q 1978, 12 (1-4), 408-25.

[27] Burki, H. J.; Roots, R.; Feinendegen, L. E.; Bond, V. P., Inactivation of mammalian cells after disintegration of 3H or 125I in cell DNA at -196 degrees C. Int J Radiat Biol Relat Stud Phys Chem Med 1973, 24 (4), 363-75.

[28] Marin, G.; Bender, M. A., Survival Kinetics of Hela S-3 Cells after Incorporation of 3h-Thymidine or 3h-Uridine. Int J Radiat Biol Relat Stud Phys Chem Med 1963, 7, 221-33.

[29] Elkind, M. M.; Sutton, H., Radiation response of mammalian cells grown in culture. 1. Repair of X-ray damage in surviving Chinese hamster cells. Radiat Res 1960, 13, 556-93.

[30] Sinclair, W. K., X-Ray-Induced Heritable Damage (Small-Colony Formation) in Cultured Mammalian Cells. Radiat Res 1964, 21, 584-611.

[31] Persaud, R.; Zhou, H.; Baker, S. E.; Hei, T. K.; Hall, E. J., Assessment of low linear energy transfer radiation-induced bystander mutagenesis in a three-dimensional culture model. Cancer Res 2005, 65 (21), 9876-82.

[32] Drew, R. M.; Painter, R. B., Action of tritiated thymidine on the clonal growth of mammalian cells. Radiat Res 1959, 11, 535-44.

[33] Drew, R. M.; Painter, R. B., Further studies on the clonal growth of HeLa S3 cells treated with tritiated thymidine. Radiat Res 1962, 16, 303-11.

[34] Keprtova, J.; Minarova, E., The effect of 3H-thymidine on the proliferation of in vitro cultured mammalian cells. Gen Physiol Biophys 1985, 4 (1), 81-92.

[35] Weizsacker, M.; Nagamune, A.; Winkelstroter, R.; Vieten, H.; Wechsler, W., Radiation and drug response of the rat glioma RG2. European journal of cancer & clinical oncology 1982, 18 (9), 891-5.

[36] Panter, H. C., Cell inactivation by tritium decays at 37 and -196 degrees C: some comparisons with X rays. Radiat Res 1981, 87 (1), 79-89.

[37] Cleaver, J. E.; Holford, R. M., Investigations into the incorporation of [3H] thymidine into DNA in L-strain cells and the formation of a pool of phosphorylated derivatives during pulse labelling. Biochim Biophys Acta 1965, 103 (4), 654-71.

[38] Banaz-Yasar, F.; Lennartz, K.; Winterhager, E.; Gellhaus, A., Radiation-induced bystander effects in malignant trophoblast cells are independent from gap junctional communication. J Cell Biochem 2008, 103 (1), 149-61.

[39] Mothersill, C. E.; Moriarty, M. J.; Seymour, C. B., Radiotherapy and the potential exploitation of bystander effects. Int J Radiat Oncol Biol Phys 2004, 58 (2), 575-9

[40] Denault C.M., Liber H.L.; The Effects of Hypoxia and Cysteamine on X-Ray Mutagenesis in Human Cells: I. Dose Response and Southern

Blot Analysis of Induced Mutants Radiation Research 1993, 135, 98-107.

[41] Little, J. B.; Hahn, G. M.; Frindel, E.; Tubiana, M., Repair of potentially lethal radiation damage in vitro and in vivo. Radiology 1973, 106 (3), 689-94.

[42] Rabi T, Bishayee A. d-Limonene sensitizes docetaxel-induced cytotoxicity in human prostate cancer cells: Generation of reactive oxygen species and induction of apoptosis J Carcinog. 2009; 8: 9. Published online May 21, 2009. doi: 10.4103/1477-3163.51368).

[43] http://ori.hhs.gov/education/products/RIandImages/guidelines/guideline.html

[44] Bishayee A, Waghray A, Barnes KF, Mbimba T, Bhatia D, Chatterjee M, Darvesh AS. Suppression of the inflammatory cascade is implicated in resveratrol chemoprevention of experimental hepatocarcinogenesis. Pharm Res. 27:1080-91, 2010.

[45] Bishayee A, Barnes KF, Bhatia D, Darvesh AS, Carroll RT. Resveratrol suppresses oxidative stress and inflammatory response indiethylnitrosamine-initiated rat hepatocarcinogenesis. Cancer Prev Res 3:753-63, 2010.

[46] Bishayee A, Bhatia D, Thoppil RJ, Darvesh AS, Nevo E, Lansky EP.Pomegranate-mediated chemoprevention of experimental hepatocarcinogenesis involves Nrf2-regulated antioxidant mechanisms. Carcinogenesis. 32:888-96, 2011

[47] Bishayee A, Thoppil RJ, Darvesh AS, Ohanyan V, Meszaros JG, Bhatia D.Pomegranate phytoconstituents blunt the inflammatory cascade in a chemically induced rodent model of hepatocellular carcinogenesis. J Nutr Biochem. 2:178-87, 2013

[48] Bishayee A, Thoppil RJ, Mandal A, Darvesh AS, Ohanyan V, Meszaros JG, Háznagy-Radnai E, Hohmann J, Bhatia D. Black currant phytoconstituents exert chemoprevention of diethylnitrosamine-initiated hepatocarcinogenesis by suppression of the inflammatory response. Mol Carcinog. 52:304-17, 2013

[49] Mandal A, Bhatia D, Bishayee A. Simultaneous disruption of estrogen receptor and Wnt/β-catenin signaling is involved in methyl amooranin-mediated chemoprevention of mammary gland carcinogenesis in rats. Mol Cell Biochem. 384:239-50, 2013

[50] Mandal A, Bhatia D, Bishayee A. Suppression of inflammatory cascade is implicated in methyl amooranin-mediated inhibition of experimental mammary carcinogenesis. Mol Carcinog. 53:999-1010 2014

[51] Baggerly KA, Coombes KR. Deriving chemosensitivity from cell lines: Forensic bioinformatics and reproducible research in high-throughput biology Ann. Appl. Stat. 3:1309-1334, 2009

[52] McCann ML, Hudes JC, Ames BN. Unusual clustering of coefficients of variation in published articles from a medical biochemistry department in India. FASEB J 23:689-708, 2009

[53] Hill, HZ, Schiff, JA, Epstein, HT. Studies of chloroplast development in Euglena XII. Variation of ultraviolet sensitivity with extent of chloroplast development. Biophys J 6:125-34, 1966; Hill, HZ, Schiff, JA, Epstein, HT. Studies of chloroplast development in Euglena green colony formation. Biophys J 6:135-44, 1966. Hill, HZ, Epstein, HT, Schiff, JA. Studies of chloroplast development in Euglena XV. Factors influencing the decay of photoreactivability of green colony formation. Biophys J 6:373-83, 1966; Hill, HZ, Alling, DW. A model for ultraviolet and photoreactivating light effect in Euglena. Biophys J 9:347-69, 1969.

[54] Stigler, SM CSI: Mendel. American Scientist 96: 425-426, 2008

[55] Kevles, DJ The Baltimore Case. A Trial of Politics, Science, and Character. W.W. Norton & Co., New York, NY. 1998

[56] Van Noorden, R The trouble with retractions. Nature 478:26-28, 2011

[57] Martinson, BC, Anderson, MS, de Vries, R. Scientists behaving badly. Nature 435:737-738, 2005.

[58] Fang, FC, Steen RG, Casadevall, A Misconduct accounts for the majority of retracted scientific publiccations. Proc Natl Acad Sci USA 109: 17028-17033, 2013

[59] A-Marzouki, S, Evans, S. Marshall, T. Roberts, I Are these data real? Statisical methods for the detection of data fabrication in clinical trials. British Medical Journal 331: 267-270, 2005

[60] Akhtar-Danesh, A, Dehghan-Kooshkghazi, M How does correlation structure differ between real and fabricated data-sets? BMC Medical Research Methodology 3:18 2003

[61] Simonsohn U Just post it: the lesson from two cases of fabricated data detected by statistics alone. Psychological Science 24: 1875-1888 2013

[62] Hudes, ML, MCann, JC, Ames, BN Unusual clustering of coefficients of variation in published articles from a medical biochemistry department in India. The FASEB J 23:689-703 2009; Varalakshmi, P, Panneerselvam, C, Sakthisekaran, D FASEB J 23: 704-705 2009; Hudes, ML, MCann, JC, Ames, BN Part 2--- Unusual clustering of coefficients of variation in published articles from a medical biochemistry department in India. The FASEB J 23:706-8 2009

[63] Marcus, A, Oransky, I How the biggest fabricator in science got caught Yoshitaka Fujii falsified 183 papers before statistics exposed him. http://nautil.us/issue/24/error/h9w-th-biggest-fabricator-in-science-got-caught

[64] Carlisle, JB the analysis of 168 randomized controlled trials to test data integrity Anaesthesia doi:1111/j.1365-2044.2012.07128.x; Carlisle, JB, Dexter,F, Pandit, JJ, Shafer, SL,Yentis, SM Calculating the probability of random sampling for continuous variables in submitted or published randomised controlled trials Anaesthesia doi:10.1111/anae.13126 2015

[65] Trivers R, Palestis, BG, Zaatari, D Anatomy of a Fraud: Symmetry and Dance. TPZ Publishers, Antioch, CA 2009

[66] Brown, W.M., Cronk, L., Grochow, K., Jacobson, A., Liu, C.K., Popovic, Z. and Trivers, R. 2005. Dance reveals symmetry especially in young men. Nature 438: 1148-1150.

[67] Baggerly, KA, Coombes, KR Deriving chemosensitivity from cell lines: Forensic bioinformatics and reproducible research in high-throughput biology. Annals of Applied Statistics 1: 1309-1332 2009

[68] Bornmann, L, Nast, I, Daniel, H-D Do editors and referees look for signs of scientific misconduct when reviewing manuscripts? Scientometrics 77: 415-32, 2008

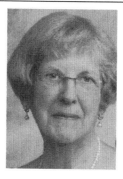

ABOUT THE AUTHOR

Helene Z. Hill, PhD, currently Professor of Radiology, Rutgers-New Jersey Medical School, Newark, researched the roles of melanin in melanoma carcinogenesis and radiation therapy resistance. She became an accidental whistle-blower in 1999 and has devoted herself ever since to tightening the oversight of and correcting the scientific record. More about her is found on her website: http://www.helenezhill.com. Email hzhill@verizon.net

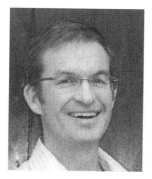

Dr John Carlisle is a specialist in anaesthesiology, intensive care and preoperative assessment, Torbay hospital, Devon, UK with main interests in long-term survival, perioperative probabilities of harm and benefit, cardiopulmonary exercise testing, and evidence-based medicine including systematic reviews. He is an editor for the journal *Anaesthesia*, was editor and author for the Cochrane Anaesthesia Review Group for 11 years. He has authored several handbooks on anaesthesia, day surgery and vascular surgery. While writing a systematic review for the Cochrane collaboration he came across the randomized controlled trials of Dr Yoshitaka Fujii and concluded that these data were fabricated. Since then, he has worked to improve the analyses of data in randomized controlled trials and tries to detect other instances of data fraud.

ACKNOWLEDGEMENTS

I want first to thank my husband who has stood by me and urged me on at every turn. Without him this book would never have been written. It was he who first noticed that the averages were appearing in Bishayee's triplicate counts at what seemed to be an unusually high frequency. And without Joel Pitt, my statistician expert when I filed for *qui tam*, this book could not have been written, for it was he who came up with the model that made it possible to calculate the probabilities that are listed in the tables. I wish also to thank the following people who have been kind enough to read the manuscript and make helpful suggestions: Charles McCutchen, a physicist at the NIH who contacted me after reading the article in *Nature* and has been helping me ever since; Clare Francis, Bart Kahr, Amy Block, Stefan Franzen fellow whistle-blowers; Brian Palestis who was kind enough to critique the manuscript and had many helpful suggestions; Robert Bauchwitz, whistle-blower and valued advisor; and all the other kind people who have put in a good word and stood behind me; most especially Margot O'Toole, standard bearer for us all.

Made in the USA
Middletown, DE
30 July 2016